THE MR PORTER PAPERBACK
VOLUME TWO

THE
MR
PORTER
PAPER-
BACK

THE MANUAL FOR
A STYLISH
LIFE

VOLUME TWO

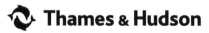
Thames & Hudson

Published in the United Kingdom in 2013 by
Thames & Hudson Ltd, 181A High Holborn, London WC1V 7QX
by arrangement with Net-A-Porter Group Ltd

British Library Cataloguing-in-Publication Data
A catalogue record for this book is available from the
British Library

ISBN 978-0-500-29127-6

Printed in China

To find out about all our publications, please visit
www.thamesandhudson.com. There you can subscribe
to our e-newsletter, browse or download our
current catalogue, and buy any titles that are in print.

CONTENTS

FOREWORD

IN VOLUME TWO OF THE MR PORTER Paperback series, our aim is to continue to inform, inspire and entertain you. There's a never-ending series of conundrums we face as a gender – whether it's choosing an age-appropriate denim jacket, which of the world's best restaurants to dine in, or how to fight off an attack from a grizzly bear (you never know when one might strike) – but we aim to make them all a whole lot easier to handle.

We like to think our advice is of the sort you'd receive from an amiable elder brother rather than an interfering colleague, and we hope you'll agree. And while some of the questions we pose and answer might appear a tad superficial – such as how to choose a Rolex or buy lingerie for a lady – most of it is of unquestionable substance: how to take the perfect penalty, for example, or nail a tie dimple. We've also thrown in a handful of interviews with men we admire – from actors and artists to tailors and fencers – as well as some appreciative essays on custom motorbikes and Italian furniture design, and some less appreciative essays on the perils of alfresco dining and commuting to work.

And underlying everything in this edition is, of course, a sense of style; something we all strive for – whether we admit it or not.

Mr Jeremy Langmead
Editor-in-Chief

"A man should look as if he had bought his clothes with intelligence, put them on with care and then forgotten all about them"

Sir Hardy Amies

THE NEW GATSBYS

*Why there'll always be millionaires who
inspire awe and suspicion*

Words by Mr John Lanchester

IF YOU HAD to reduce all 20th-century literature to a single question, that question would be: who are you? And by extension, who am I? It's a question that operates at deep philosophical levels, touching on our innermost being and sense of self. It's a question about how we describe our selfhoods, and how we process what happens to us, and who we want to be, and what are our dreams and fears, our most private needs, the things we daren't say even to ourselves. But it's also a very basic question, a question we can ask on a daily basis about anyone we might bump into: who is this guy? What's his story? Who is he pretending to be, and who is he really?

One of the reasons why *The Great Gatsby* is such an extraordinary work is that it takes this question, a question that's central to so much 20th-century writing, and turns it into the fulcrum of the story. It is, as screenwriters like to say, right on the nose. Who is Gatsby? Not just in a philosophical sense, but also in a basic and literal way: who is this guy, and where did he make his money, and what's he up to? Is he for real? We can see the outside – the money, the parties, the bling – but where did he come from? It's part of Mr F Scott Fitzgerald's genius that he shows us how exciting this question is to the world around Jay Gatsby. The people enjoying Gatsby's fabulous hospitality are turned on by wondering about the mystery behind it.

Gatsby is a modern archetype. Economic booms create Gatsbys. For all the recent difficulties, there are more rich people than there have ever been, and so there are more men like Gatsby than ever before. (I was going to say there are more people like him, but that's wrong: the Gatsby archetype is not gender-neutral. A female adventuress is a thing of wonder too, but is a different kind of human riddle.) In the past couple of decades, new categories of Gatsby came into being all around us: hedge fund Gatsbys, commodity Gatsbys, dotcom Gatsbys, start-up Gatsbys, venture capital Gatsbys and IPO Gatsbys and every other variety of man who's made so much money so fast that for the rest of us there is a kind of built-in mystery to them. Without that mystery, there's no Gatsbyism going on: these are the kind of men about whom people enjoy speculating. Exactly how was it he made that first million? It's always a faintly titillating question.

The other indispensable component for Gatsbyism is to be very good at spending money – by which I mean lavish, unconflicted, un-tortured, ambivalence-free. There is a type of very very rich person who attends to the spending of every cent as carefully as if they were very very poor. Gatsbys are the opposite of that. People are so troubled by money that there is something magical, and also troubling, about those few of us who seem not to be. Nobody understood this better than Mr Fitzgerald, and he gave this understanding to his most famous character.

If the archetype still holds truer than ever, and there are more Gatsbys than ever all around us, that doesn't mean there haven't been some changes. The most important is that the new mystery men are more international. The modern Gatsby doesn't come from the place where he now struts his stuff – if he did, people would know too much about him. The mobility of the modern international rich is one of the most striking things about them. It's a mobility which parallels that of modern capital. The capital, which can go anywhere, goes to the place which is friendliest to it, and the people do the same thing. Contributing to this unprecedented mobility is the fact that the signifiers of super-wealth are now so international. The brands are the same everywhere you go; they speak the same language.

In terms of a tax regime's friendliness to international wealth, no great city beats London; add the ideal time zone and the language, and it's no mystery why London is the global centre of Gatsbyism. But the idea that place is important is a little misleading. Gatsbys live not in a place but in Gatsbystan, which might be in the sixth arrondissement, or Greenwich Village, or Knightsbridge, or their yacht. Just as it's not quite clear where they are from, it's also not quite clear where they live – in more than one place, for sure. Wherever there's a Gatsby, there's a string of empty properties somewhere else. There's also a party, and plenty of attractive people, and a whiff of mystery, and a sense that many of the people present are wondering exactly where and how all this ends.

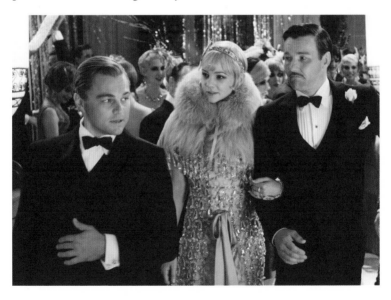

FROM LEFT: Mr Leonardo DiCaprio, Ms Carey Mulligan and Mr Joel Edgerton in Mr Baz Luhrmann's 2013 adaptation of *The Great Gatsby*

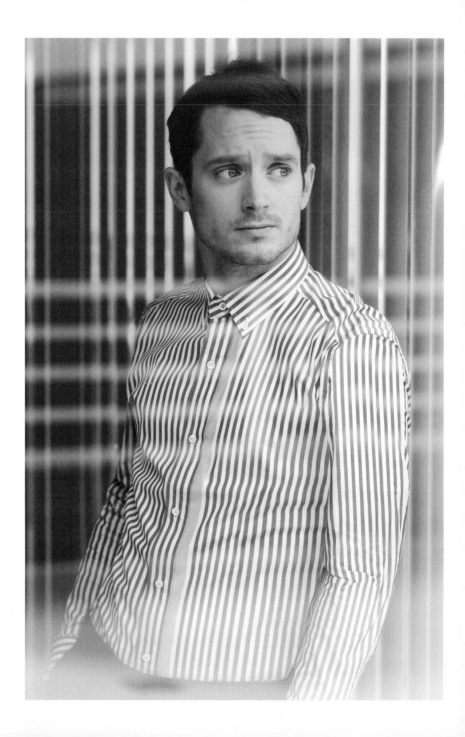

MR ELIJAH WOOD

*The talented actor – who's portrayed everything from hobbits
to psychos – talks about movies, music and maniacs*

Words by Mr Mike Hodgkinson

WHEN IT COMES to cinema, Mr Elijah Wood is a card-carrying internationalist. "Predominantly, the movies that I love the most these days are being made in Europe or Mexico or Asia," he tells MR PORTER over coffee, on a clinically bright Los Angeles morning. "A fair amount of incredible film-makers have come out of Spain in the past five to 10 years. I just worked with two Spanish film-makers on their English-language debuts [Mr Eugenio Mira, *Grand Piano*; and Mr Nacho Vigalondo, *Open Windows*]. And I was recently in Japan, talking to some film buyers there. There are some incredible film-makers in Japan too."

We're at a French café near Venice Beach, a suitably cosmopolitan venue given Mr Wood's love of the unusual and the foreign. Fresh from trips to the Far East and the Iberian Peninsula, the actor who cemented his legend with *The Lord of the Rings* movies (shot in New Zealand) holds strong claims to world-citizen status. He's a resident Angeleno who has extended his horizons beyond Hollywood in all directions. Resisting the temptation to rest on his mainstream Middle-Earthen laurels, Mr Wood has embraced global film culture, pursuing a diverse slate of projects in multiple countries, as both an actor and producer.

Speaking of his involvement in 2012's *Maniac,* a movie from that most visceral and controversial of sub-genres – gore – he says:

5

"The thing about this particular *Maniac* film is that it's a stylised version of the original." He played the mother-fixated psycho in a remake of the 1980 grindhouse landmark. The film is directed by Mr Franck Khalfoun, who rang the changes by making explicit an admiration of Italian *giallo* legend Mr Dario Argento – one of splatter cinema's most revered stylists – and shot the entire movie from the killer's point of view.

"The original had its own sense of style I think, but it was pretty dirty. I wouldn't even classify it as a B-movie," says Mr Wood. "I'm not a huge fan of remakes, especially horror-film remakes. But I was intrigued by this. What resulted was far more stylistic and beautiful than I had anticipated. It was initially pitched to me as: you'll play the killer, and you'll only be seen in reflections. So interesting. And each sequence effectively is a single shot, so every scene became this puzzle of trying to figure out how I was involved, where the camera moved. It was like a dance."

Cinematic horror is no casual dalliance for Mr Wood, who has established The Woodshed, a production company that is specific to the genre. In 2013, Mr Wood filmed *A Girl Walks Home Alone at Night* – an Iranian vampire Western, shot in black and white, and performed entirely in Farsi. Also on The Woodshed's portfolio is *Cooties*, the product of an unlikely script collaboration between Messrs Leigh Whannell (*Saw*) and Ian Brennan (*Glee*). "It's a horror comedy about a zombie-like affliction that affects children at school."

Throughout our chat, Mr Wood is enthusiastic and engaging, apparently relishing the freedom to hatch an assortment of creative plans on the back of his success with the *Rings* movies. He looks like a man at ease with himself, and this comes across in a relaxed approach to personal style that walks the line between knowingly unforced and truly unconcerned. "Yeah, I suppose fashion is a part of my life. Not in any kind of major way. I think everybody has a costume – I'm pretty simple. I just like things that are relatively classic and timeless."

He reveals that he doesn't go shopping often, but makes an exception when he visits Japan. "For me, fit has everything to do with it. In Japan, every single thing I put on would fit, which just does not happen in the US. I kind of go a little crazy. It's nice to go into a store, see something I like and go, 'That will fit'. It's awesome. Japan's a great place to shop."

How about shopping online? "I checked out MR PORTER for the first time recently. It's amazing. The selection of designers is one of the largest I've ever seen from any one source, from new up-and-coming designers to really established lines. Very cool."

The thing that links all of Mr Wood's exploits and interests is his willingness to take in the big picture, an approach that also surfaces on the sidelines of his career, in music. "I listen to everything. Some of the labels that I most love are primarily reissue labels, such as Now-Again Records, Finders Keepers out of the UK, and Light In The Attic Records – they do full reissues of specific albums, but they also put out really wonderful compilations of world and psychedelic music."

Simian Records, the music label Mr Wood founded in 2005, is "sort of in flux at the moment", and he also still enjoys to DJ on occasion (vinyl rather than digital – "it's far more satisfying"). "I spend more time digging back than I do looking into what's happening currently. I find it more gratifying – I think it's harder now to find really great records that you fall in love with. It's far easier to find something from the past that blows your mind."

This antique disposition also surfaces in Mr Wood's love of Los Angeles architecture. In 2012, he campaigned to save a 51-year-old taco stand from the wrecking ball – "We have so little history as it is in Los Angeles and I think it's important we preserve it" – and cites City Hall and the 2nd Street Tunnel as favourite local structures. From turn-of-the-century craftsman homes in Pasadena, the Victorian mansions of Angelino Heights and the now-razed neighbourhood of Bunker Hill, preserved only as a film noir memory in movies such as *Criss Cross*, he's an admirer of them all.

"There was actually a building here in Venice, a very small craftsman bungalow. Ray Bradbury had lived there when he was writing *The Martian Chronicles*. The new owners tore it down. It broke my heart."

Mr Wood takes a last, wistful sip of coffee.

"But I feel as if the tide is changing. I feel as if people are more aware of our history, and what little of it we have left."

And with that he's off, bags packed, ready to carve out some history of his own.

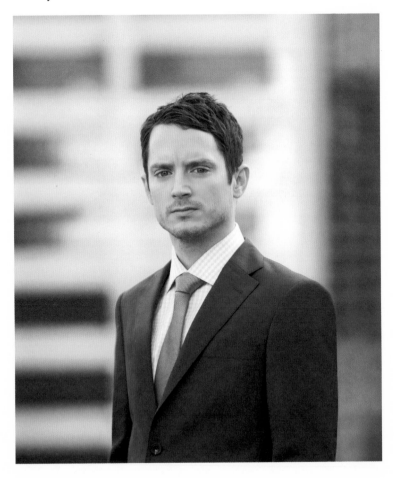

FASTEN YOUR SEAT BELT

The commute to work is fraught with danger –
from fellow travellers and your conscience

Words by Mr Alex Bilmes, editor of British *Esquire*

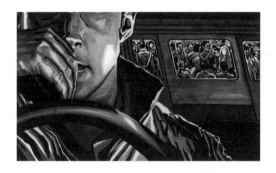

GENTLEMEN, fasten your seat belts: what I am about to admit is so deeply, mortifyingly uncool that frequently, in conversation, I lie about it, to hide my own shame and avoid the righteous indignation of those less fortunate and more enlightened than me. Deep breath. Here goes. My name is Alex Bilmes and I drive to work. Yes, in a car. To central London from, well, not very far at all outside central London. Takes about 25 minutes, door to car park, on a good day. Twice that or more when they're digging up the roads. And when are they not digging up the roads? So call it closer to an hour, each way, in a big, heavy, diesel-gobbling, Arctic-ice-sheet-shrinking, family-man, four-wheel-drive estate vehicle.

A tank-like German one with room for about 17, plus pets and surfboard. Most days there's only one person on board (minus pets and surfboard). And me – a mere slip of a thing!

Please understand, I haven't always done this. For the preceding two decades, I was on the bus and the underground with the rest of the right-minded world. But then I got my current gig, and with it came said parking space underneath Soho, and after two decades in the tunnels and on the top deck, I couldn't resist. Seriously: could you?

This new way of travelling between home and office by car has been an interesting exercise in learning how the other faction lives – sometimes a freewheelingly gratifying exercise; at other moments knuckle-whiteningly frustrating.

It has also offered some perspective on my years as a schlubbish, publically transported commuter.

Driving to work has its ups and, inevitably, its downs. To the bedraggled man waiting at the bus stop in the rain, I might seem the definition of the pampered executive. But fellow members of the motorcade will know that while it's an advantage being warm and dry, it's less fun being stuck in snarl-ups, gesticulated at by van drivers, despised by pedestrians and spied on by police cameras. Driving is, paradoxically, both more comfortable and more stressful than walking, or running, or pedalling, or hopping on a bus or a train.

Herewith, then, are some observations.

I

Driving to work makes you stupider. OK, I'm pretty up on current affairs, courtesy of the BBC's teeth-grindingly irritating *Today* programme, which blasts on my Blaupunkt each morning. But I no longer read novels, or serious non-fiction, except in bed. Believe me, I've tried balancing Ms Zadie Smith on my steering column in light-to-medium traffic, but she kept falling off. I tried Mr Michael Lewis, too, but cyclists were getting in the way, and I began to fear prosecution if I hit one.

Driving to work makes you more successful but less interesting, because you can spend the whole time on your hands-free, Bluetooth-enabled mobile phone chatting up clients, impressing bosses and admonishing staff, thereby actually starting and finishing work about an hour earlier and another hour later than Tube and subway users. Driving is no longer about indulging in me time. You're alone but not alone. As opposed to on the Tube where you're not alone but alone. Which brings me to...

3

Driving to work is lonelier. Yes, it's a relief not having one's face jammed into another straphanger's armpit at 7.45 in the morning, somewhere deep beneath Bayswater or the Brooklyn Bridge. But on the flip side, there are no chance meetings with old friends or silent flirtations with alluring strangers. If Mr Michael Fassbender's sex addict character in *Shame* had driven to work, even he would never have got laid. As for *Mad Men*'s Pete Campbell, forget about it.

4

Driving to work means never again earwigging on strangers' conversations. And while the tinny noise pollution of a teenager's iPhone earbuds is hardly the breakfast birdsong we might ideally expect to start our days with, life in the city really isn't life in the city unless you're rubbing along with and even up against your fellow urbanites. Strangely, perhaps, I miss the *esprit de corps* of the communal commute. Stuck in my car, separated from the hustle and bustle, I may as well be working in the provinces. And that, my friends, is not a fate I'd wish on my enemies.

5

Driving to work is, for all the annoyances of two-mile-an-hour London traffic, more physically comfortable. Especially if your car has massage seats. Oh, yes.

6

Even massage seats can't disguise the fact that driving to work is no less stressful than being stuck on the 7.20 to St Pancras or waiting for the Number 94 only to discover you've lost your travel pass at the precise moment it finally turns up. In fact, many is the day when, like Mr Michael Douglas' D-Fens in *Falling Down* – the best film ever made about the fear and loathing of driving to work – I frequently feel like abandoning my vehicle in the middle of the gridlocked highway, taking my pump-action from its hiding place underneath my seat and striding through the city randomly taking people out. Sorry, but I do.

7

On days when I don't feel murderous – they do come along occasionally – driving to work adds a considerable burden of responsibility to my mornings and evenings. It's not just that I don't have an excuse for being late when the Victoria line goes down. It's that suddenly the lives of all the other many road users – old ladies, schoolchildren, people in electric wheelchairs – are in my hands. The vigilance required to get to work and back without killing one of these specimens, the lightning reactions and Mr-Ryan-Gosling-in-*Drive*-style avoidance tactics necessary to prevent that inconvenient eventuality, is really quite astonishing. Especially when I've had a drink. Which brings me to...

8

Alcohol. When you drive to and from work, you have to monitor your booze intake. When I say monitor I mean: you can no longer drink until you get home. Which means you feel better in the morning, but you never have fun again. Not just that but...

9

...If you have an after-hours work function to attend, people will ask you for a lift home and get quite huffy when you refuse (because the last thing you want to become is a taxi service for slurry-breathed work colleagues).

10

What with London's congestion charge, the parking fines, the traffic violations and the incredible cost of fuel, servicing and repairs, you need to be a billionaire to drive to work. I'm not a billionaire. This whole thing is unsustainable. And yet, and yet... I've got the car and I've got the space. Might as well use them. Right?

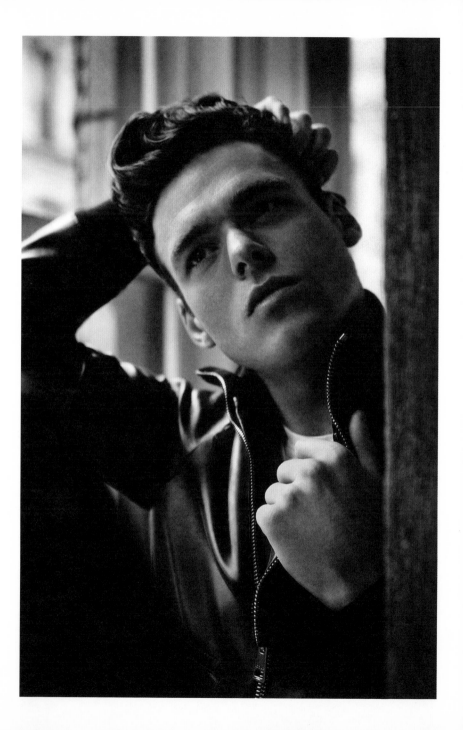

MR RICHARD MADDEN

The Game of Thrones *actor is set to emerge from the*
gore of the HBO series with his head held high

Words by Mr Jeremy Langmead, Editor-in-Chief, MR PORTER

MR RICHARD MADDEN is beginning to get recognised quite a lot. At a private party in Claridge's, London, I watched a 50-year-old man ask if he could photograph Mr Madden and his co-star Mr Kit Harington, for his "14-year-old niece; she's a big fan of the show". As if. That photo was totally taken for his own pleasure: the gentleman couldn't hide his delight that he was in Mayfair with the show's two lead characters, Robb Stark and Jon Snow.

Game of Thrones – a cross between Middle Earth and *The Sopranos* – is massive. The cult novels by Mr George RR Martin have been dramatised by HBO with no expense spared on gore, full-on arse-banging sex and eye-popping locations. And this has given Mr Madden, who has been critically acclaimed for his theatre roles in London's West End (including *Be Near Me* with Mr Ian McDiarmid) and the BBC TV dramas *Worried About the Boy* and *Birdsong*, a whole new level of fame.

And it looks as though the talented Scot's notoriety is only going to get bigger. Starring in movies with the likes of Ms Rebecca Hall and Ms Cate Blanchett – Mr Madden is playing Prince Charming alongside Ms Blanchett in Sir Kenneth Branagh's *Cinderella* remake – he can barely contain his excitement. Talented, handsome and with absurd levels of energy, he's in New York for a few days' holiday. However, before the craziness truly kicks in, he is enjoying the city. Shopping is high up on his agenda – burnished suede Chelsea boots from Prada, a cashmere peacoat from J.Crew – as are cocktails. Mr Madden likes cocktails; in fact, Mr Madden likes anything that takes place at night. He's one of those people who comes alive in front of a camera, or at a party; both seem to energise him. At a small soiree MR PORTER throws in the Empire Suite of the Standard High Line hotel, the day after the photoshoot, Mr Madden eases into the role of unofficial co-host; he greets the guests, plies them with Martinis and conversation, and relishes every moment of it: his eyes darting around for mischief and merriment. Despite a jet-lagged host (me) and the fact that it's only a Tuesday night, the party finishes at around 4.30am. At 6pm the following evening, as I'm beginning to wilt at my desk, Mr Madden is texting from the bar at the Bowery Hotel suggesting a Ketel One and soda might be just what I need. It turns out he's right.

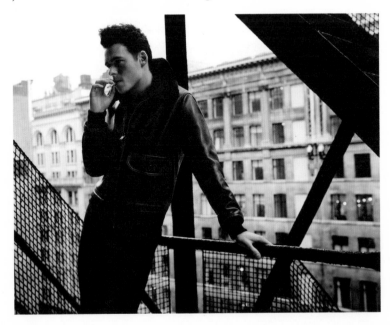

THE RULES OF MODERN DATING

As your age rises, so do the stakes.
One fortysomething single writer explains…

Words by Mr Simon Mills

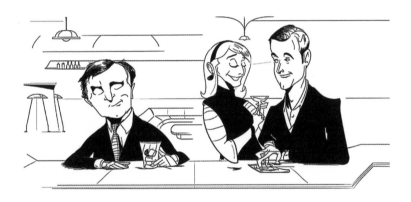

THE BEST dating movie in recent history was 2011's *Crazy Stupid Love*, mainly because it stars the unassailably sexy, thinking man's dream triumvirate of Mses Julianne Moore, Emma Stone and Marisa Tomei. But also because Mr Ryan Gosling's Jacob Palmer, a sharply dressed, smooth-talking, bar-flying serial shagger offers a series of refreshingly accurate lessons in modern-day dating to Mr Steve Carell's clueless, tongue-tied, recently separated, slope-shouldered, emotionally broken fortysomething, Cal Weaver. The segment about the two male leads' wildly disparate approach to wardrobes is particularly well observed.

While Mr Gosling's cruising attire is styled for results – even at the mall, *even while eating a slice of pizza* – Mr Carell's character has seriously let himself go, all the way into Silicon Valley territory. "Are you Steve Jobs?" asks Mr Gosling, incredulously. "Are you the billionaire owner of Apple computers? No? Then you have no right to wear New Balance sneakers. Ever." A high-tempo shopping montage ensues, in which Mr Gosling forces his hapless middle-aged project to invest in a capsule wardrobe of contemporary dating *schmatta*. Mr Carell winces at the designer prices. "Be better than the GAP," says Mr Gosling. "Say it."

A single man's clothes, dating clothes, are not just for dressing; they are carefully executed gift wrapping, a visual CV that trumps up sartorial proficiency and alludes to bank balance, taste, a wider aesthetic, career choice, worldliness and confidence. Make no mistake, every detail will be noticed, dissected and forensically appraised by your date just moments after your entrance. This is dating *CSI*, baby – and you, my single friend, are the "vic". So, during that first encounter you want her to see your best bits and disregard your imperfections. You want clothing that slims, enhances, elongates and sexifies, not just insulates.

Make tailoring your friend. Ditch anything loose, oversized, baggy, sloppy, avuncular and/or daddish. Wear items that encourage confident, upright deportment. Keep tones dark and sober. Maintain a palette of muted, classy colours: navy, petrol blue, black, white, grey, and so on. If you go for jeans, opt for indigo blue, with a selvedge, and fitted as if for an urban rodeo. Footwear? Proper bench-made shoes, please. Never opt for sneakers on a date. She'll think you are one of those unemployed sorts with a PlayStation problem.

Best to lie up when asked your age, but to dress seven to 10 years younger. If you are, say, 45, think 37 with your cut of trouser. If you are wearing a suit, definitely lay off the pinstripes. This is a date, remember, not a sales pitch. (And, while we're at it, your mobile phone number handwritten on a napkin – replete with playful flirty message – is much sexier than proffering a business card detailing your direct line at the office.)

Just before you leave the house, look at yourself in a full-length mirror and cast a cruelly critical eye over your ensemble and ask yourself: if you walked into a bar and bumped into you, would you like to take you home? If the answer is anything as positive as "maybe", then you are ready to hail a cab.

Now comes the tricky bit: talking. It's worth noting that Mr Gosling's best chat-up line in *Crazy Stupid Love* was, after a female had said she didn't know what she was doing tonight, "That's OK, I do." And as lines go, it is a pretty slick one. Crucially, because it came out of Mr Gosling's mouth. And not yours. The truth is that actors, fictional characters and rock stars tend to have an unfair advantage over us civilians. Their celebrity is, in effect, an opening gambit in itself, so there is no need to lay on the cheese. Don't believe me? Here are the favoured, apparently fail-safe opening lines reportedly employed by two well-known swordsmen.

Mr Rod Stewart: "Hello darlin', what have you got in that handbag?" (he apparently used this to chat up Ms Rachel Hunter). Sir Mick Jagger: "Hello, I'm Mick." The last one being the most effective, especially if you happen to be Sir Mick, of course.

But if you don't happen to be an A-list superstar, being funny, cheeky and gently audacious is always a winner. Even if it's civilian you, trying to nail a celeb. I lunched with the pillowy-lipped supermodel Ms Rosie Huntington-Whiteley recently and she told me that (pre-Mr Jason Statham) she'd been very nearly seduced by a guy in a bar who had a moustache tactically tattooed on his forefinger. When he caught Ms Huntington-Whiteley looking at him across the room, the handsome boy raised his inked digit to his upper lip and waggled it. With that goofy move, the stranger came this close to pulling a Victoria's Secret Angel. If only he'd known.

That said, any seasoned singleton will tell you that venue is more important than ink or vernacular. Regard everywhere you go (with the possible exception of work) with priapic potential. Hunting grounds such as nightclubs and cocktail bars are OK when you are in your twenties, but cougars and DILFs prowl parks, supermarkets, cinema multiplexes, service stations, weddings and middle-class family dinners. Contact may be made by swings and sandpits. At checkout queues and butcher counters. ("Hello darlin', what have you got in that trolley?") After initial contact, send a pithy, funny, grammatically correct and spell-checked text message minutes after your brief encounter (when you have vacated the venue) suggesting a second meeting.

Once you go out for dinner (for which you will be picking up the bill and paying for the taxi afterwards), she'll be liking your intellect and goofiness in equal measures. Be urbane, informed and a very, very good listener. You should be subtly, sexually driven, but not salivating for it. So don't ogle, because you'll just look incredibly desperate.

Be miserly with the compliments (let's face it, if she's pretty, she'll have heard them all before), but make the ones you do deliver thoughtful, memorable and truly devastating. If it's a first date, whatever you do, don't touch her. Instead, pay rapt attention to everything she says, no matter how annoying and silly it might be. Nod in approval and be sympathetic and understanding. You should know that it is quite possible to endure a whole evening with a first date without her asking you a single thing about your own career and personal life. You have to learn to not be surprised or offended by this.

However, when you get the chance, make it very clear that sex – maybe even a relationship and babies – is what you eventually want from her. You don't want to go on three expensive dates, having invested in some nice clothes and put aside your beloved New Balance sneakers to suddenly have her announce that you have become her "friend", now do you?

THE MAGIC OF MOTORCYCLES

A round-up of timeless rides that continue to surpass the rest

Words by Mr Donnie Little

THERE IS something about motorcycles. Transcending class and status like no other form of transport, you can turn up anywhere with a motorcycle helmet under your arm and you've already made a statement. What that statement is depends on you and the bike you choose to ride. Here is a small selection of machines we believe say all the right things…

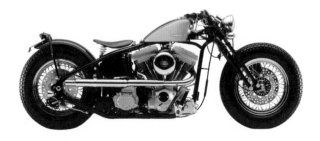

ZERO ENGINEERING TYPE 5 EVO

Hand-built, knee-high and to many a minimalist masterpiece, the Zero Engineering Type 5 is the brainchild of Japanese custom bike builder Mr Shinya Kimura. Made using a rigid gooseneck frame and 1940s-style springer forks, it oozes the kind of credibility that makes other riders and passers-by stop and stare.

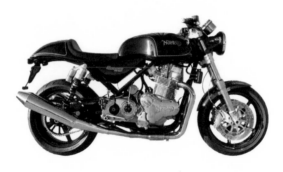

THE NORTON COMMANDO 961

This Norton has the ideal blend of power, torque and handling to make every trip eventful without being terrifying, and the looks, prestige and exclusivity to cause a fuss when you stop for fuel. If you want retro racer cool with an illustrious name and modern handling, performance and reliability, then this is the bike for you.

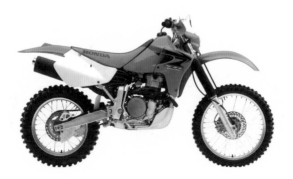

HONDA XR650R

As proven to those that have seen Mr Ryan Gosling riding a Honda XR650R in *The Place Beyond the Pines*, the single-cylinder dual-sport machine is as happy robbing banks as it is ploughing through mud. For law abiders like us, though, the long-travel suspension and lofty riding position would make light work of the daily commute.

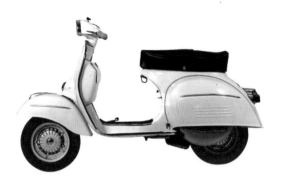

VESPA SS180

With its "step-through" design that protects the rider from both the elements and the oily moving parts, the Vespa is easily the coolest way to traverse the modern metropolis. Our model of choice? The 1964-1965 SS180. Sprightly enough to do battle in the urban sprawl yet with the classic lines that helped Vespa define the 1960s.

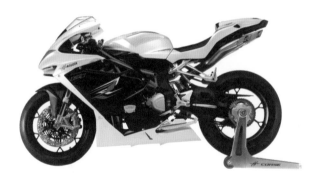

MV AGUSTA F4 1000 RR

There are those for whom only the latest, fastest and most extreme machine will do, and the most recent is undoubtedly the MV Agusta F4 RR. Even with sophisticated software reining in nigh on 200bhp, the RR is a brutal and unforgiving motorcycle that will have you questioning your skills and sanity – in a good way.

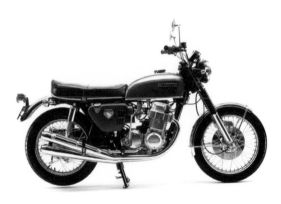

HONDA CB750K

The CB750 made its debut at the end of the 1960s. Boasting four cylinders, four exhausts, 8,500rpm and front disc brakes – features usually reserved for race bikes – it offered something revolutionary. The result? Here was a bike that was stylish, reliable and oil-tight – and the first to be recognised as a superbike.

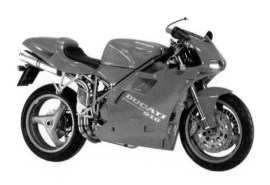

DUCATI 916

Upon launch in 1994 the Ducati 916 caused a sensation. The Mr Massimo Tamburini-designed lines were futuristic yet timeless, the under-seat exhausts and single-sided swingarm were both practical yet beautiful. Massive torque and sublime handling made it unique. Even today, the Ducati 916 is a thrilling motorcycle.

ART OF THE ROBE

The iconic nightwear item that is as elegant as it is practical

Words by Mr Jeffrey Podolsky

I HAVE many an important and historical relic from my late father: his vast collection of invaluable pipes; his 70-year-old pearl-handled razor blade; his first editions of *Catcher in the Rye* and Mr TS Eliot's *Collected Poems*; along with 60-year-old LPs of recordings of Messrs Eliot, WH Auden, Dylan Thomas and Tennessee Williams. My father, an insomniac, would listen to these throughout the night while alternating between Churchillian Havana cigars and his pipes, and sipping Armagnac from a snifter in his wood-panelled library.

From among all the irreproducible clothing he bequeathed me (including three-piece tweed suits of such precious swatches that they'd be hard to replicate at even the most revered Savile Row tailor today), it is his robe I cherish most of all. Purchased in Italy, it is cut from a super-fine silk, in a deep burgundy and blue paisley, and still bears its label from the early 1950s: "Arbiter, Lori & Mari, Via Condotti, Rome" – and, also, in Italian, "Made in Spoleto".

It would be unimaginable for my father or men of his era not to don a robe when rising from their beds. It not only served practical purposes in terms of keeping them suitably warm on frigid evenings, but there was also an unspoken elegance to its importance in their wardrobe. It was the polite thing to wear – no one wanted to appear in front of the live-in help in their PJs or, heaven forbid, their boxer shorts. In that less artificially harried day when one didn't check their emails in the morning before greeting their wife, lover, or children, the robe was the essence of chic casual dress within one's home, worn both in the morning and evening over their nightwear – or in my father's case, a pair of white Indian cotton pyjamas with blue piping from Brooks Brothers.

Changing into such an ensemble in the early evening signalled to his own psyche that the working day was done and it was indeed time to relax, whether reading in front of the fire or writing a letter to friends.

The elegance and practicality of the robe has become something of a long-lost art in men's style and dressing. In an age when most of us are obsessed with accoutrements and accessories, we should rediscover our genetic roots and realise that the robe is not just an accessory, but a way of living.

Even the thought of fetching the newspapers outside my apartment door while in only a pair of boxers is a worrying prospect, and undoubtedly a far more horrifying sight to my neighbours. As such I've carried on the tradition of wearing a robe, so well illustrated in the films of Messrs Clark Gable and David Niven, sometimes to a lover's horror, but always to my personal delight. I may well wake up alone most mornings – the only staff to witness my sartorial statement being my rescued mutt and her young puppy – but I feel infinitely better in terms of my own segue into the day after donning my father's robe and reading the morning news over an espresso.

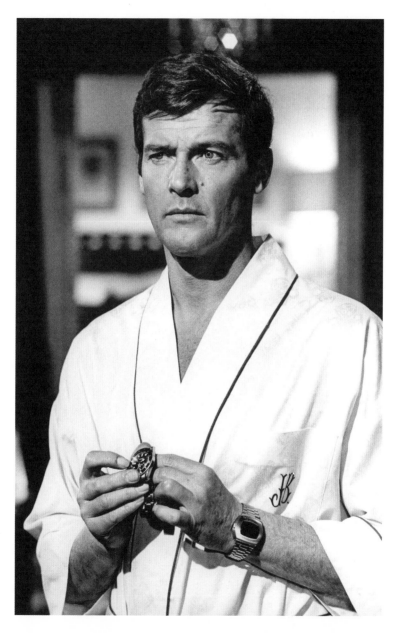

Sir Roger Moore in *Live and Let Die*, 1973

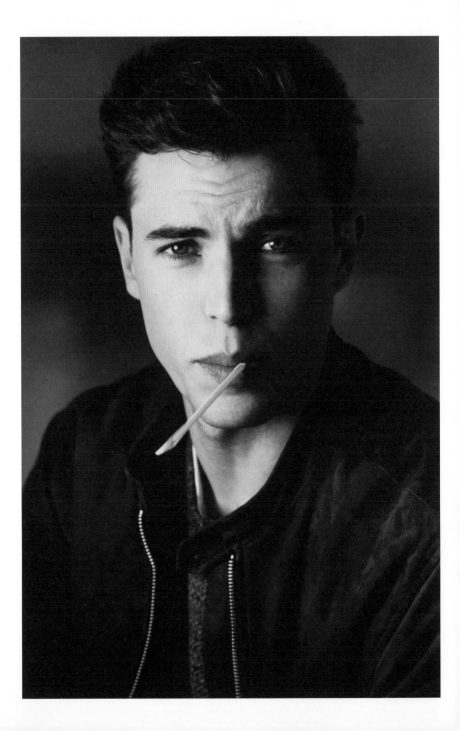

MR TOM HUGHES

The handsome and talented British actor reveals
he has another string to his bow

Words by Mr Chris Elvidge, Senior Copywriter, MR PORTER

"I WAS FACE DOWN in the mud," laughs Mr Tom Hughes as he describes his stint at an SAS training base for his movie, *I Am Soldier*, while buttoning up for his shoot with MR PORTER.

These are busy times for the British actor, hotly in demand after starring in two well-received, high-profile shows. First came *Dancing on the Edge*, a five-part series directed by Mr Stephen Poliakoff, which followed the fortunes of a black jazz band in Depression-era London, and shortly after came *The Lady Vanishes*, a lavish adaptation of the book that inspired the classic Sir Alfred Hitchcock thriller of the same name. And while these roles have seen his profile rapidly rise, it seems that success was always on the cards for him. Mr Ricky Gervais, on casting him in one of his very first roles in 2010's *Cemetery Junction*, described him as "a rock star and a film star who embodies the spirit of Liam Gallagher, Richard Ashcroft and James Dean".

A graduate of London's prestigious Royal Academy of Dramatic Art, Mr Hughes hardly had time to find his feet before being picked up by Burberry to star in one of its campaigns. "When they asked me if I'd be interested, I'd been out of drama school for about six months," he says. "I had no press. This was before *Cemetery*

Junction – nothing that I'd filmed had even come out yet. My agent asked, 'How do you know who he is? How do you even know that he exists?' Their response was, and I quote, 'We are not at liberty to disclose our sources'."

"I must have sold my soul to the devil," he adds with a grin – despite the fact that it's plain to see, with his enviable looks, that no such Faustian pact would have been necessary.

Eager to avoid the "actor-cum-model" label, Mr Hughes is quick to play down his modelling experience as just that: an experience. "Fashion's a world I really know nothing about," he says. "I was so green, I had no idea what I was doing. Douglas [Booth] and Emma [Watson] were there, and Tom Guinness, too – I just followed their lead. I didn't even know the photographer. I had no idea who Mario Testino was; why should I? He's not a guitarist, is he?"

Moving away from the topic of fashion, his coyness quickly dissipates. He speaks with a passion about music, describing it, alongside acting, as one of his two driving forces, and the first of the two to exert an influence on his life. "I started playing guitar when I was six years old. That's before I first knew that I wanted to be an actor," he explains, adding that, "the two have always gone together – one seems less vibrant without the other. It comes from the fact, I think, that they're both about the same thing – a desire to tell stories."

And with music playing such an important role in his life, can we expect it to blossom in a similar way to his acting career? "I've been meaning to get in the studio," he says. "I've got something like 150 songs running around in my head, and I just want to see some of them put down on record. Creativity isn't just about having these thoughts, it's about acting on them, too, and turning them into something tangible."

THE CLASSICS

DENIM JACKETS

Since this rugged American classic never goes out
of style, here are four ways to wear it well

Words by Mr Peter Henderson,
Senior Fashion Writer, MR PORTER

THE APPEAL of the denim jacket is greater than the sum of its parts. Sure, it's practical (lightweight yet rugged; warm but breathable) and is constructed from the iconic material originating from either 19th-century Genoa or Nîmes (depending on which etymology you follow). But what gives the denim jacket its edge – and ensures it will always remain in our wardrobes – is its cultural associations. At its roots the denim jacket is straight from a Steinbeck novel: invented as utility wear, it speaks of the hard work and salt-of-the-earth honesty associated with the 19th- and early 20th-century US ranchers, railroad workers and gold rushers who wore them. A few decades later, advertisers would immortalise this essence in the Marlboro Man, a fictional Everyman character (who often sported a denim jacket) whose purpose was to rid filtered cigarettes of their "effeminate" image. In the second half of the 20th century, the denim jacket became indelibly associated with popular culture as it was adopted by artists, Beat intellectuals, rock stars, punks, bikers and hip-hop stars. These days, designers produce denim jackets that remain true to their roots while having the level of quality and finishing that we have come to expect in our clothes.

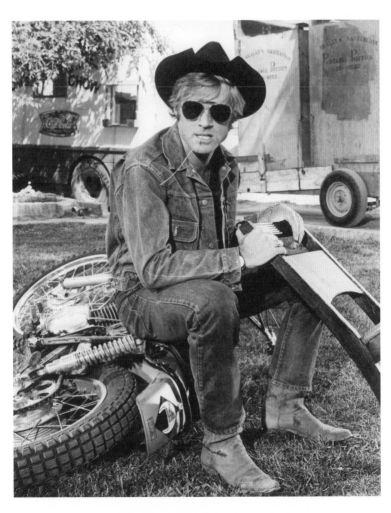

Mr Robert Redford in a film still of
Little Fauss and Big Halsy, 1970

Seen here on the set of *Little Fauss and Big Halsy* in 1970,
Mr Robert Redford's hybrid biker-cowboy look is effortlessly
stylish – and provides evidence that double-denim can work
very well.

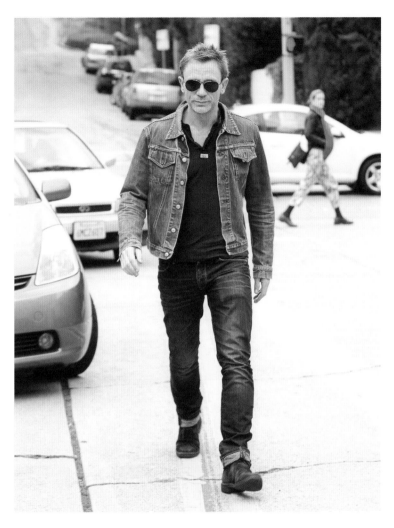

Mr Daniel Craig out and about in LA, 2011

Photographed in Los Angeles in 2011, Mr Daniel Craig's workwear-inspired casual outfit is easy to emulate for an effortless off-duty look. Note how his denim jacket is lighter than his jeans and Henley T-shirt.

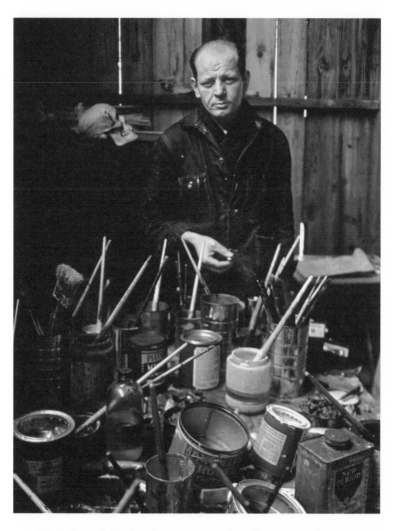

Mr Jackson Pollock in his Long Island studio, New York, 1949

Abstract expressionist painters, including Messrs Willem de Kooning and Jackson Pollock, wore denim jackets and overalls as an unofficial uniform. Even if you're not an artist, a judiciously applied splatter of paint can add a certain something.

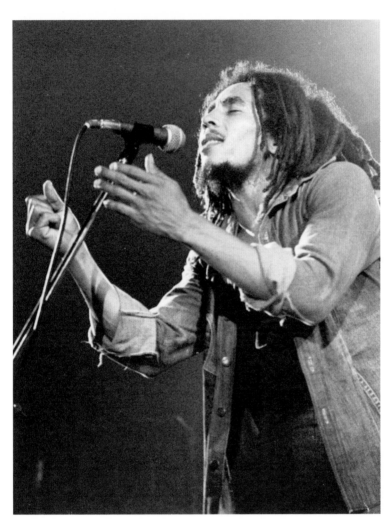

Mr Bob Marley performs with the Wailers
in Voorburg, Holland, 1976

Mr Bob Marley often wore a denim over-shirt or jacket for
performing. Despite its rugged heritage, the denim jacket works
well for a more Bohemian aesthetic too.

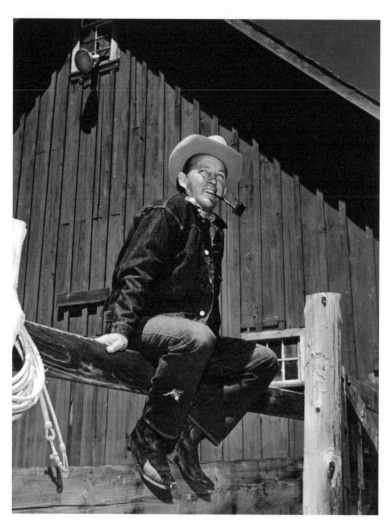

Mr Bing Crosby perches on a farmyard fence, circa 1955

Mr Bing Crosby wore immaculate tailoring for performing but favoured denim jackets off duty. In the 1950s he was refused entry to an upscale hotel for wearing a denim jacket, prompting Levi's to create him a bespoke denim tuxedo.

I

You can wear a denim jacket with denim jeans, provided they are
of different colours or washes. Generally speaking, it looks best if
your jeans are darker than your jacket.

2

For a modern, preppy look, slip on a denim jacket in place of
a blazer with an Oxford shirt and slim knitted tie.

3

In winter, consider wearing a denim jacket as an extra layer
underneath an overcoat (in place of, say, a cardigan). Pop the collar
of the denim jacket (but not the overcoat) and you'll instantly look
like a fashion editor attending the menswear shows.

4

The denim jacket is inherently casual, so you shouldn't look stiff
wearing one. Roll up the sleeves and don't be afraid to rough it up. If
you purchase a raw (unwashed) denim one, it will need breaking in.

5

The fit should be snug in the body and arms. Baggy, blousy denim
jackets were big in the 1980s, but this is no longer the case.

6

A denim jacket with a simple white T-shirt is a fail-safe option.

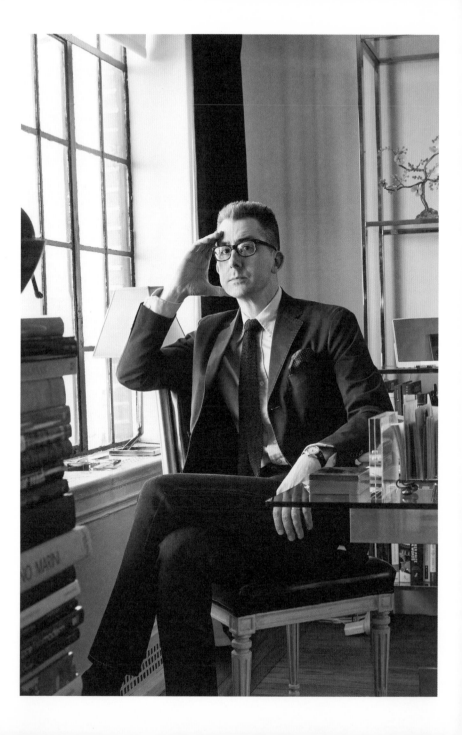

MR MICHAEL HAINEY

In his New York apartment, US G Q's deputy editor opens up about his intriguing family memoir, After Visiting Friends

Words by Mr John Ortved

WHEN US *GQ*'s deputy editor Mr Michael Hainey was six years old, he woke up to discover that his father – a night-time copy editor at the *Chicago Sun-Times* – was dead. *After Visiting Friends: A Son's Story,* a memoir Mr Hainey took 10 years to complete, is not only a touching remembrance, but something of a potboiler, as the seasoned journalist searches out medical records, police reports, old friends and estranged family members – taking us back to Chicago in the 1960s, into a world of hardboiled newspaper men – to discover what really happened to his father on the night of his death.

In he and his partner Ms Brooke Cundiff's homey, stylish West Village apartment, Mr Hainey sat down with MR PORTER to discuss the power of poetry, sequels and good reporting.

Now that your book is edited, published and on the bookshelves, do you feel some closure?
I think there's a sense of resolution. But, we as children are our parents' sequels, in terms of stories. We are created by our parents, but our stories and their stories are so intertwined. I know what happened. But it doesn't mean I stop thinking about him. I think

I'll always have that "What if he lived?" question. There's closure to the mystery, but I don't think that wound ever heals.

It's not just a memoir; it's also kind of a mystery.
I've always wanted to be a poet. That's how I started writing. That's why the lines are very compressed. Poetry teaches you to sort of crystallise your thinking. But I never saw it as a mystery. I was writing a book that was a search for an answer. I didn't realise until I had finished, and when people were giving me feedback, that it's a mystery.

You write about your mother and father's first date, and she's wearing a blue skirt and a yellow cashmere cardigan. These are intimate details that make this book feel real. How did you get those details?
That's what stays at the heart of the book: reporting. The book opens with a scene in which my grandmother says, "There's lots of stories you've never heard." It's a book where there are stories inside of stories, inside of stories. And good stories have details. I also wanted to pay homage in the book to the power of memory – how people can remember details that are so vibrant for them, and yet you never really learn them unless you ask them.

Your mother raised two boys on her own.
With this book, I went looking for my father but I found my mother. She is the hero of this book, but – I've always told people – she's the hero of my life. Back in the 1970s there weren't many single women living in the suburbs. I was the only one in my school who did not have a father. People weren't even divorced in my neighbourhood. I also forget she was 33 when he died. So she's incredibly strong.

Your father, a reporter, made it a point to dress well. Here you are, deputy editor of GQ. Do you think there's a sartorial line we can draw as well as a journalistic one?

It was surprising when my grandmother told me that detail. I guess maybe it's one of those things I inherited, but I never would have known about it.

.

The news business is always in the background. Your dad and his friends, the papers in Chicago in the 1960s all clustered together downtown. Media is so, so different now. It seems much less clubby.
Anyone who looks at it has to say, wow, that must have been a fun time. I would have liked to experience what they had. But half of the guys – they drank, they smoked – didn't make it to 60 because of that.

You came to journalism through Spy magazine.
Spy was the most amazing finishing school. I came there to be exposed to the great minds: Graydon Carter, Kurt Andersen, Susan Morrison. There was a group of us that were young assistants and reporters and writers, getting paid nothing. There was a place downtown with $5 pitchers of beer. What meant a lot to me was coming up with nothing, and you sort of make your way in New York. It's sort of funny now – I see 25-year-olds talking about having dinner at RedFarm – and I'm like, "Where do you get the money to eat at these restaurants?" I marvel, "So you have $4.50 to get Starbucks every morning?" I don't want to sound like the old man but I'm amazed, it now seems to be about consuming the culture.

Your book has excellent placement at our neighbourhood bookstore, Three Lives & Company.
My editor emailed me and wanted to know if I would come by Three Lives and sign copies, and I said "Sure". As Brooke and I turned the corner, we saw it in the window. I was talking to the owner, Toby, and I started to cry. I said, "I worked on this book for 10 years – my studio was over there – I would walk by your bookstore. I would look in the window and I would think, 'One day I will be here'."

When you were younger – because your father died before he was 35 – did you just assume you were going to die young?

Yeah. I can remember being nine or 10 and thinking, what's the point of having a family? What's the point of falling in love? I will die and I will leave people behind. It's pretty grim for a boy. But, as I got to be 33, 34, 35, and came out the other side, I had to really think and find out what I wanted to do. As I was coming up on that age that he died, that kind of precipitated wanting to find out the truth. It all coalesced on that. I never thought I'd outlive him.

In the book, you go so deep, personally and professionally. As a journalist reading After Visiting Friends, *it's like what it must be for a comic watching Mr Louis CK. You're watching the process. You really went down and dirty.*

I think the book resonates with people because there's a fair amount of me saying, "I don't know, I'm lost, I'm confused." This is a very personal story, but it's also universal, because we all have family, and every family has a secret, or secrets. And we all want to find the answers. I wanted to inspire people. I thought it was important to show the reader that this was not an easy thing. But I hope I can inspire people by showing I did this. I stuck with it. I was afraid. I had doubts and fears. But my journey could be your journey.

I WISH I WAS THERE

10 magical sporting moments we'd have loved a ringside seat for

Words by Mr Dan Davies, editor of *Esquire Weekly*

WHAT ARE THE CRITERIA for choosing a list of the sporting events we wish we'd been at? Well, the first has surely got to be the quality of the sport on show. It is all very well getting tickets for the Super Bowl, a heavyweight title bout or World Cup final, but if the action fails to live up to the import of its setting then what advantage has been gained over those watching at home on television?

The factors taken into consideration in deciding this list – which can, by its very essence, be nothing less than subjective – include historical significance and how such performances or encounters defined what came before and after, the willingness of the protagonists to push themselves beyond the limits of what they previously believed possible and, last but not least, the buttock-clenching drama of the feats on show.

Sport has the ability to transcend, transform and inspire. It can also bind people together, however briefly, in a common purpose. But as any sports fan will tell you, the most important aspect for the lucky few that get to witness such exploits is the cache of being able to say you were there.

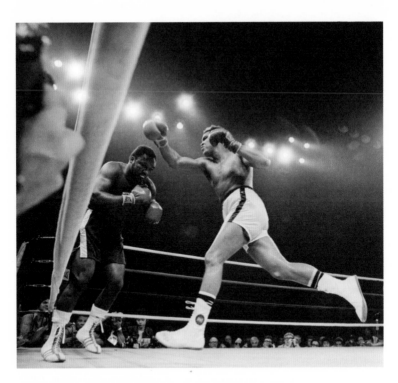

"THRILLA IN MANILA"
MR MUHAMMAD ALI VS MR JOE FRAZIER
1 October 1975

Mr Joe Frazier won their first fight in New York in 1971, and three years later Mr Muhammad Ali gained his revenge. But when these two great heavyweights met for the final time, six miles outside of Manila in the Philippines, they were fighting for more than the world championship. According to American sportswriter Mr Jerry Izenberg, "They were fighting for the heavyweight championship of each other." In a match of vastly contrasting styles and personalities, Mr Frazier's motivation was to silence an adversary who had mocked him mercilessly, but after 14 punishing rounds his trainer decided his man could take no more. Although victorious, Mr Ali said it was the closest he'd come to death.

MR FRANKIE DETTORI'S "MAGNIFICENT SEVEN"
28 September 1996

"I could have an each-way chance in the first, and I may win the third," said Italian jockey Mr Frankie Dettori on race morning in Ascot, England. Two wins would have been a fine return, but to win all seven was considered impossible. That verdict hadn't changed even when he rode to victory in the first three races. But when Mr Dettori won the next three, the bookmakers were facing potentially ruinous losses. When he romped home in the seventh race of the day, it changed the lives of those on both sides of the ledgers.

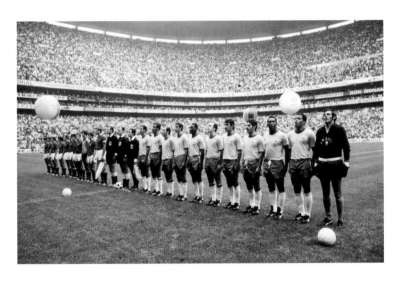

MEXICO WORLD CUP FINAL – BRAZIL VS ITALY
21 June 1970

The 1970 World Cup in Mexico witnessed the flowering of arguably the greatest international football team of all time. Brazil, led by Mr Carlos Alberto and featuring Messrs Pelé, Rivelino and Tostão, faced Italy in the final, with both nations bidding for a third title.

Pelé opened the scoring with a spring-heeled leap and downward header. Italy equalised before Brazil cut loose in the second half with goals from Messrs Gérson, Jairzinho and a strike for the ages from Mr Alberto after a sublime display of passing and individual skill.

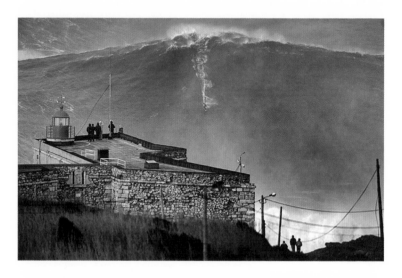

MR GARRETT MCNAMARA BREAKS THE RECORD
FOR THE LARGEST WAVE EVER SURFED
28 January 2013

The weather on the coast of Nazaré, just north of Lisbon in Portugal, looked dire, but to big wave surfer Mr Garrett McNamara it was perfect: a combination of strong winds and a high tide promised monster waves. At 8am the Hawaiian entered the water, and after a frustrating wait the swirling mists cleared. Mr McNamara spotted two huge waves but chose to ignore them on the educated hunch that a third, bigger one, would be rolling in behind them. He was right. "It was like looking down from the top of a giant mountain," Mr McNamara says of the moment he first surveyed the 100ft wall of water he would ride on his way to a place in the record books.

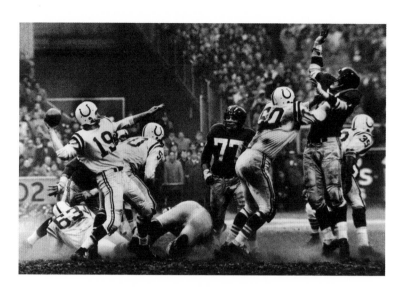

BALTIMORE COLTS VS NEW YORK GIANTS
28 December 1958

In late 1958, 64,000 spectators packed into the Yankee Stadium in New York to watch the Baltimore Colts beat the New York Giants in an encounter described as the greatest football game ever played. Two late touchdowns gave the Giants a 17-14 lead but a field goal by Mr Steve Myhra with seven seconds remaining sent the game into overtime. Driven by their legendary quarterback Mr Johnny Unitas, the Colts scored the clinching touchdown when Mr Alan Ameche launched himself into the end zone to win the first NFL Championship game to be decided in sudden death. The sporting landscape of the US was altered forever.

BRITISH GRAND PRIX
— MR BARRY SHEENE VS MR KENNY ROBERTS
14 July 1979

The UK's Mr Barry Sheene and the US' Mr Kenny Roberts were fierce rivals who had traded world titles in the two years before they took to Silverstone in 1979. The Londoner burst from the start line with a wheelie on his Suzuki before the race settled into a thrilling bout of thrust and parry, with his nemesis on a Yamaha. At one stage Mr Sheene flicked a V-sign at Mr Roberts as he pulled ahead. But at the end of the race it was the American who edged past on the final lap. "We were rivals," said Mr Roberts after Mr Sheene succumbed to cancer in 2003. "I simply did not want him to beat me at any time, and he felt the same way about me."

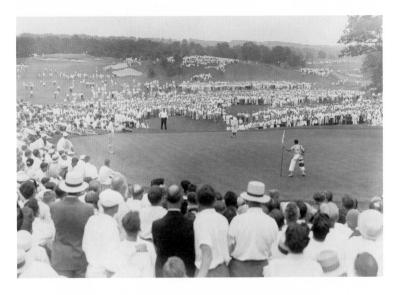

MR BOBBY JONES WINS THE GRAND SLAM
27 September 1930

Against a backdrop of the Great Depression, an amateur from Georgia, US, achieved a feat that has never been equalled: winning all four of golf's major championships in the same year. When Mr Bobby Jones won the British Amateur Championship and the Open Championship, it was described as the greatest achievement in golfing history. It earned him a ticker-tape reception along Broadway on his return, but Mr Jones, who had backed himself with a bookmakers at odds of 50-1, went on to win the US Open. He then completed the "impregnable quadrilateral" by winning the US Amateur. He promptly announced his retirement, aged just 28.

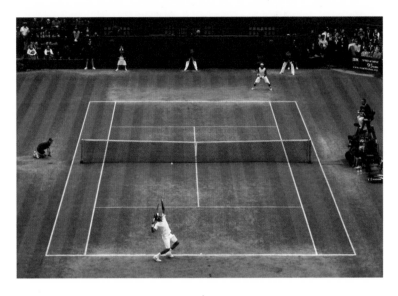

WIMBLEDON MEN'S SINGLES FINAL
— MR RAFAEL NADAL VS MR ROGER FEDERER
6 July 2008

Mr Roger Federer was bidding to become the first man to win six consecutive Wimbledon men's singles titles; Mr Rafael Nadal was aiming to be the first since Mr Björn Borg in 1980 to win the French Open and Wimbledon back to back. Mr Nadal, defeated by his Swiss rival in the previous two finals at the All-England Club in London, won the first two sets before rain interrupted the third. When the skies cleared, Mr Federer claimed the third set on a tiebreak, and repeated the trick in the fourth, saving two Championship points with outrageous winners. The deciding set finally went to Mr Nadal 9-7, sealing victory after what, at four hours and 48 minutes, had been the longest Wimbledon final in history.

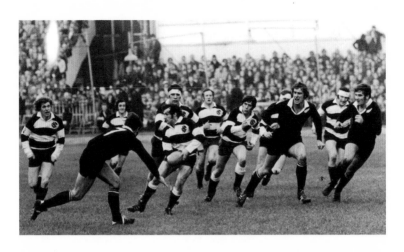

BARBARIANS VS NEW ZEALAND ALL BLACKS
27 January 1973

Two years after the British and Irish Lions became the first
touring side to beat the All Blacks in a Test series in New Zealand,
the fabled southern hemisphere rugby team were still smarting.
Now, in the 22nd match of their 1973 tour of Britain, in which
they had only lost three matches and remained unbeaten in Tests
against Wales, Scotland, England and Ireland, the Kiwis faced the
Barbarians at Cardiff Arms Park. Only a few minutes in to the
game they eventually won by 23-11, Welsh fly-half Mr Phil Bennett
gathered the ball and unleashed a series of sidesteps that launched
a move that swept the length of the field and resulted in the greatest
try in the history of rugby union, scored by Mr Gareth Edwards.

MR JESSE OWENS AT THE BERLIN OLYMPICS
3 and 4 August 1936

On 3 August 1936 in Berlin, a modest 22-year-old American made
a mockery of Adolf Hitler's theories of Aryan racial superiority
by winning the Olympic 100m final. The next day he claimed
the long jump gold medal before embarking on a lap of honour

with the great German hope Mr Luz Long. Mr Owens went on to win gold in the 200m and 4x100m relay and, despite the Nazi backdrop, was mobbed by the German people wherever he went. "After all the stories about Hitler, I couldn't ride in the front of the bus," Mr Owens later said of his return to the US. "I had to go to the back door… I wasn't invited to shake hands with Hitler but I wasn't invited to the White House to shake hands with the president either."

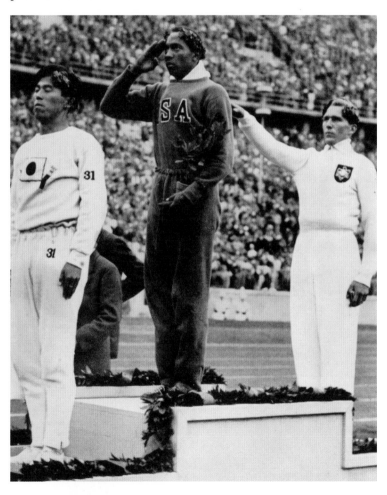

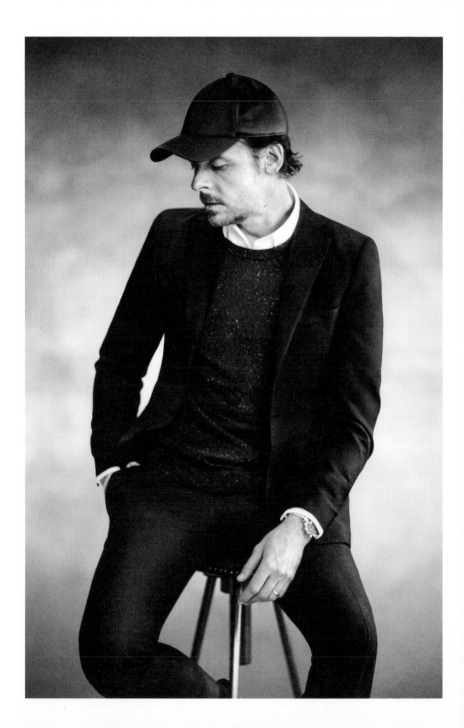

THE LOOK
MR SIMON PEGG

The British actor reveals why, after Star Trek Into Darkness,
he boldly took his career to The World's End

Words by Mr Alex Bilmes, editor of British *Esquire*

LET'S START, as he would wish us to, with a spoiler alert: those
hoping for anguished confessions of moral impropriety, diva-ish
hysterics or mumbling Method actor pretentiousness should seek
out celebrity interviews other than this one. Very sorry to report,
but Mr Simon Pegg really is, as advertised, a thoroughly decent
bloke – smart, funny, down-to-earth, self-deprecating without
a hint of false modesty – who also happens to be a crucial part of
no less than three thriving Hollywood blockbuster series. These
include *Star Trek*; *Mission: Impossible* and *Tintin*. Hold on, there's
actually a fourth recurring credit to his name: Mr Pegg is also the
voice of a one-eyed weasel in the megabucks *Ice Age* animations.

And these are just the supporting actor projects that keep him
busy when he's not pursuing his proper career, as the co-writer and
star of charming, funny, irreverent comedies including *Shaun of the
Dead* (zombies terrorise North London), *Hot Fuzz* (*Bad Boys* shoot
up the English shires) and his third film, in what he and director
Mr Edgar Wright call their "Cornetto Trilogy": *The World's End*,
in which a provincial pub crawl takes on apocalyptic dimensions.

Before that, in 2013, Mr Pegg got to pull on the Starfleet crew
neck for the second time as Scotty, the geeky chief engineer
("Dilithium chambers at maximum, Captain!"), in *Star Trek*

Into Darkness, high-flying director Mr JJ Abrams' sequel to the 2009 monster hit that breathed bodacious new life into what had become rather crumbly characters and scenarios. While at the helm of the *Star Trek* franchise, Mr Abrams also announced in 2013 that he would be directing the seventh *Star Wars* movie.

And *Star Wars* is really where Mr Pegg came in, as the co-creator and leading man in *Spaced*, the Channel 4 comedy in which he played a *Star Wars* obsessive not entirely unlike himself; Mr Pegg's university dissertation was not, as is often reported, specifically about *Star Wars*. That said, "It was about the social implications of popular cinema of the 1970s, so *Star Wars* came into it."

All of which means not only can he speak intelligently about the significance of both Stars *Trek* and *Wars* – and quote Baudrillard on the infantilism of society while doing so – but also he has a vested interest in both franchises. As the following comments testify: "My immediate reaction [when hearing that Mr Abrams was to direct the next *Star Wars*] was to say to him, 'Don't forget *Star Trek*, will you?' He said to me, 'Absolutely not', and I trust him implicitly. I love him as a director and a person, so it was extremely exciting news. And when I discovered that the old cast could be back – you know, Harrison Ford [who played Han Solo] and Mark Hamill [Luke Skywalker] – it's as if the sequels that we always wanted and not those bloated f**king soulless pieces of shit that..." He trails off, still as angry about Mr George Lucas' interminable *Phantom Menace* and its follow-ups as if he'd first seen them yesterday.

He's passionate about science fiction, then, but that's to be expected. Mr Pegg, so the narrative goes, is the archetypal sci-fi geek who, thanks to a mysterious cosmic accident, has been beamed from his modest West Country origins – dad a jazz musician, mum a civil servant – onto planet Hollywood, where the natives have somehow mistaken him for one of their own.

It has to be said he didn't do much to diminish this impression by calling his autobiography *Nerd Do Well*. But, I suggest to him, it's still a somewhat reductive reading of his story. He's a successful professional with a substantial track record as a writer and performer: why should he not have just as much right as his buff American co-stars to appear in these big-budget enterprises?

"I think it's just that the irony of events is never lost on me," Mr Pegg says, explaining his public profile as our man in space, the Everyfan who lucked out. "In order to remain uncynical and to enjoy life I try to see everything from the point of view of my seven-year-old self. And if my seven-year-old self had been told he was going to be in *Star Trek*, he would have been amazed! A lot of people try to play it cool, they take it in their stride, but I work in a job that I absolutely love and I never want to take it for granted."

Married to Ms Maureen McCann, a former music A&R, since 2005 – and they now have a young daughter, Matilda – Mr Pegg lives just outside of London and seems almost entirely unaffected by his celebrity: a resolutely well-adjusted man in a world unhealthily preoccupied with the behaviour of famous people. How come he's not more unpleasant?

"There's a great quote," he says, "at the end of a documentary called *Overnight*, about an overnight success. It says, 'Fame doesn't turn you into an arsehole, it just brings out the arsehole you always were.' And I can see why famous people become arseholes because you are treated with an immense amount of... care. But that's simply because as actors we are the cosmetic face of every project, so it's very important that we get where we're supposed to be on time, we look how we're supposed to look, because if we don't then someone will lose money. So we're constantly handled. And if you start believing that you're handled because you somehow deserve it then you turn into an arsehole. I've got enough people around me that would tell me if I was becoming a bit of an idiot."

Mr Pegg is firm on this point, as he is on many points. He is a highly entertaining conversationalist, a good-natured ranter, with all sorts of theories on all sorts of things.

Pernicious celebrity culture was born, he says, because of home video cameras, which "completely demythologised the idea of being on television, so the auspiciousness of celebrity started to disappear." Happily, of course, like all true satirists, he offers not just the critique of the industry and its spawn, but the cure, in the form of his own more personal projects.

Unlike its predecessors, Mr Pegg says, which were both homages to US genre movies, *The World's End* is indebted, if anything, to the social science fictions of Mr John Wyndham, the English novelist of creepy mid-century classics *The Day of the Triffids* and *The Midwich Cuckoos*, among others. It's about a group of old friends, in their early forties, who reunite 20 years after a legendary pub crawl around their English town, to do it all over again. Its cast includes Mr Pegg, his regular sidekick Mr Nick Frost, as well as Messrs Paddy Considine, Martin Freeman, Eddie Marsan and Ms Rosamund Pike.

"It came from Edgar and me talking about the idea of going back to where you're from and it not being the same as you left it. It is about male friendships, and it's about growing up, getting older. It's probably the most serious film we've ever made, but I also think it's the funniest because it's really silly, too."

Meanwhile, Mr Pegg being Mr Pegg, he's keeping himself busy with other things, too. In 2013 alone he made a pilot for a US TV crime series called *Lost Angels*, in which he plays a Jewish stand-up comedian in 1940s LA, as well as taking the lead role in the film *Hector and the Search for Happiness*, alongside Ms Pike again.

He's not doing much to dispel the geek-done-good storyline, is he? "No," he says, "but I'm thankful we've got our own stuff as well because that's formed the backbone of it all and that's what's given us a calling card and introduced us to people such as JJ, Spielberg and John Landis. I feel very lucky to get to work with them, because they are the people who inspired me when I was growing up."

And with that he's off to boldly go where no unassuming Gloucestershire pop culture obsessive has gone before. Impossible – and a bit churlish – not to wish him luck, so I do.

STANDOUT SHIRTS

Seven reasons why a tropical take
on print is making a comeback

Words by Mr Peter Henderson, Senior Fashion Writer, MR PORTER

Bold, printed shirts are seeing a revival. That's right: the standout shirt is back. But hang on a minute. Before you order that piña colada and head for the pool, there are a few things to bear in mind. The look is in no way related to your uncle Ernest's Caribbean cruise outfits, nor to Mr Tom Selleck's somewhat seedy *Magnum P.I.* attire. Vibrant shirts may be in, but that doesn't mean good taste is out. For starters, anything featuring scantily-clad hula girls is out of the question, ditto those printed with maps or resort names. Equally unappealing are shiny silk printed shirts. It's about innovative patterns printed onto tailored, well-made shirts.

MR PORTER'S GUIDE TO THE STANDOUT SHIRT

I

Unless you're ready to make a real statement, a bold patterned shirt calls for the rest of your outfit to be relatively plain. Offset vibrant prints against solid block colours and simple shapes. Chinos, unstructured blazers and jeans with minimal detailing work well.

2

Most standout shirts look best untucked, however those cut like formal shirts can be worn tucked into tailored trousers for a sharp, mod-inspired look.

3

Similarly, ties should be avoided unless the shirt is cut in a more formal way, with a structured collar and substantial cuffs. And if you do go for a tie, make it a slim, dark knitted or woven one – a standard silk tie looks too lustrous against a lively pattern.

4

If you want to tone things down a bit, consider wearing a standout shirt underneath a sweater with just the collar and cuffs visible.

5

Unless you live in Hawaii, where "Aloha Fridays" are the norm, reserve your most vivacious printed shirts for your downtime and not for the office.

6

Bear in mind that bright prints are not particularly forgiving to very pale skin or to excess baggage around the waist.

7

However extravagant the print, it's vital to wear the shirt with a devil-may-care attitude.

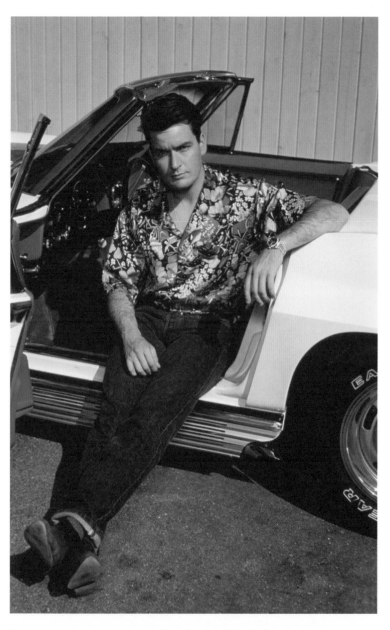

Mr Charlie Sheen takes a break in California, 1991

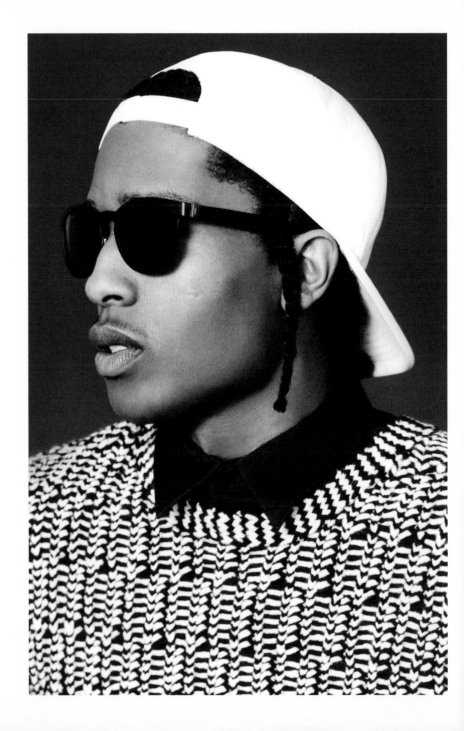

THE LOOK
A$AP ROCKY

In MR PORTER's exclusive interview, the
platinum-selling hip-hop artist reveals all

Words by Mr Mansel Fletcher, Features Editor, MR PORTER

IT'S ONLY A SHORT distance from the tough streets of Harlem to the front row of a New York fashion week runway show, but it's a journey that few rappers have made. A$AP Rocky, however, managed it even before the release of his No.1 debut album, *Long. Live.A$AP.* His appearance at Paris fashion week in January 2013, dressed in clothes by British designer Shaun Samson, reinforced the impression that he has come a long way from a childhood that inspired the line on his album's title track, "I thought I'd probably die in prison". On meeting A$AP it becomes obvious that if any rapper is going to transcend hip-hop's cultural ghetto it's him, despite the fact that he has admitted to dealing drugs in the past. Lots of MCs enjoy enough success to make the leap, but few take the opportunity. Yet the way A$AP explains it, he makes it sounds so simple: "I realised the streets were my reality, and I wanted to make another home, so I started doing positive things. Some people have it in them to get out, and some people are content to stay in the hood. You'd be kind of stupid to get stuck in a bad predicament your whole life, but I feel blessed because I know where I came from and everything I've been through."

That "everything" includes two family tragedies. The first was the death of his older brother, Ricky. "He was a gang-banger, a Blood [member], and he got killed. I wanted to be like him, but when he died on the streets I realised that the streets are not the place I wanted to make home," he remembers. His older brother didn't just inspire A$AP to escape the block; he gave him the tools to do so by introducing him to rap music. "My brother was a hip-hop fan, and when I was eight he made me rap for the first time – he was beating on the table to make a beat, I started rapping and he encouraged me to keep doing it." Much more recently A$AP also lost his father. "My dad passed in 2012," he explains. "I'm just getting over it. I couldn't cry because I was so hurt. He caught pneumonia on a Friday and died on the Sunday, so it was unexpected, but at least he got to see me do this." His father was also a rap fan: A$AP's real name is Mr Rakim Mayers, his Christian name inspired by the 1980s rapper behind *Paid in Full* and "Eric B. is President".

Central to A$AP's success is that his take on rap music is Pan-American. Since it first emerged from the parks of New York's Bronx, hip-hop has always been rabidly territorial. In the 1980s rappers from the five New York boroughs battled over the culture's geographical origins, while in the 1990s a rivalry between the US east and west coasts cost the lives of rappers Biggie Smalls and Mr Tupac Shakur. A$AP is different, in that his taste, and his sound, cover the gamut of hip-hop culture. When asked about his influences he mentions Southern rappers Geto Boys and Three 6 Mafia, Midwesterners Bone Thugs-N-Harmony, LA's Dr Dre, and New York's Ruff Ryders label. No wonder his breakthrough song, "Purple Swag", with its woozy production, is so hard to geographically pin down. This could be the result of the way that the internet enables people to abandon tribal loyalties and take a pick-and-mix approach to music, or, as *The New York Times* suggested in a story about A$AP's friend and collaborator, A$AP Yams, the result of a rather considered approach to marketing. I'd tend towards the former given A$AP Rocky's ease with the once-heretical idea of a New York rapper enjoying music from the west coast and the "Dirty South". "I don't know if it was wrong [to enjoy music from all over America]," he says, "but I can say that my brother used to do it, so I adopted it." His taste in clothes is also unusual given his profession. On the track "Peso", which he released in August 2011, A$AP declares that it's "Raf Simons, Rick Owens, usually what I'm dressed in". The line immediately suggests a sophisticated taste in style, something he reveals goes back to 2005. "At eight I started getting into fashion, brands such as Tommy Hilfiger, Nautica and Ralph Lauren," he remembers. "But in 2005 I started wearing John Richmond jeans. I was into Prada and Dolce & Gabbana at the time and that's why I started to wear tight jeans, because I wanted to be a model. I started to do freelance work for Calvin Klein, so it just stuck."

A$AP arrives at the MR PORTER shoot wearing clothes by Jil Sander, Balenciaga and Junya Watanabe, but, again breaking the rap mould, says he has no plans to set up his own fashion brand. "It would be disrespectful to take my stardom and bully my way into the fashion industry, because I didn't go to [fashion] school to learn about design, sketching and fabrics. I just enjoy it; I'm a consumer." Given the macho nature of the hip-hop world I obliquely ask if A$AP's interest in fashion, and the cut of his jeans, have ever led people to call his masculinity into question. He responds bluntly: "People say I'm gay sometimes, but I have a lot of bitches so why would I care? It doesn't bother me at all. You know why they say that? Because they can't say that I suck, they can't say that I'm not handsome, and they can't say that my lyrics are wack, so they say that I'm gay because they don't have anything on me." Another way A$AP sets himself apart is by eschewing the bling aesthetic. He admits to owning a nice watch, but that's it. "I have a Rolex, but no diamonds. Rappers wear diamonds to compensate for a lack of fashion sense. I don't even have pierced ears – I'm not into that, it's too much." No less extraordinary is his taste in cars. "I'm into vintage cars – there's a Jaguar E-Type in the 'Goldie' video." He believes his taste is part of the appeal of his crew, the A$AP Mob. "I'm not your average rapper. For us to be thugs and admire high fashion is kind of odd, but people like it."

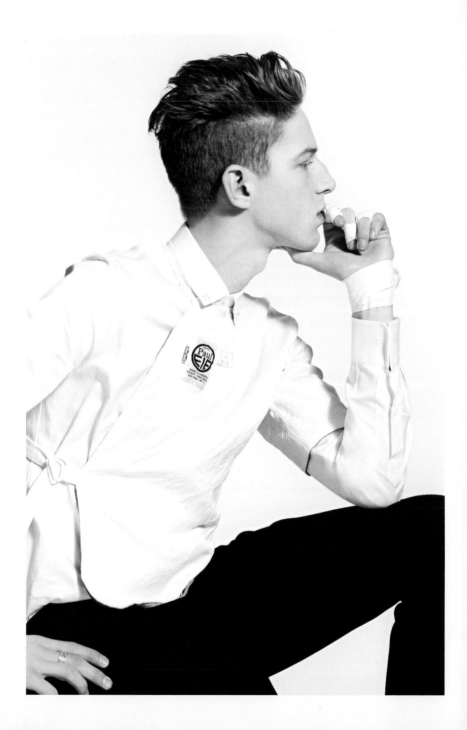

ONE TO WATCH

MR RACE IMBODEN

The Olympic fencer reveals why fashion is the perfect
foil to the pressures of his sport

Words by Mr William Van Meter

"IN FENCING, the pressure is on you," says Olympian swordsman turned model Mr Race Imboden. "It's all mental. You have to think of exactly what to do or you will lose. With modelling you just listen and do what you're told. It's actually a refreshing change."

Mr Imboden, who has an eye-catching tattoo of the Olympic rings on his arm, didn't embark on a modelling career from being scouted on the street. An agent at Re:Quest Model Management saw him on television when he competed with the US team in the London Games. "The next thing you know, I was on runways," he says. "My first show was Duckie Brown. And then that season I did Marc by Marc Jacobs and it rolled from there." Yes, he sees the incongruity in his two career paths. But fencing, in many ways, did prepare him for his second career. "They don't relate to each other that much," he admits. "But when they told me, 'Oh with modelling you're going to have to travel so much, life will be crazy', I was like 'meh...' – I've been travelling overseas by myself since I was 14. I was never at school. I was never there. I was travelling all the time. That was my high-school experience. I missed my prom. My life was always in a different country every week."

Besides his strawberry blond hair, the most standout feature of Mr Imboden is probably his rather regal nose. "I got into a skating accident when I was little," he says. "That's what made it crooked. I definitely had my period where I was like, 'Oh man I've got such a big nose', but I'm used to it now." Sitting on a bench outside a coffee shop in Williamsburg, Brooklyn, he is wearing a colourful Pendleton coat over black jeans, and a crisp denim jacket and vintage brown rugged hiking boots. It's a considered look in anyone's book. He is, in fact, so well put together one would assume he is rocking gifted gear from various fashion gigs.

"It's not!" he protests. "This is the one day I'm not wearing my free fashion week clothing! I like to wear Pendleton, but I also like moodier, all-black New Yorker type of clothing."

Born in Tampa, Florida, but living in Brooklyn from a young age, fencing quickly became the focal point of Mr Imboden's life in his new city. "I really started training when I came to New York," he says. "We moved right across the street from a fencing club."

He has big plans for the coming years, with aims to study business and work in the music industry. Right now though, it's modelling that has both him, and his parents, excited. "My mum is super into it," he says, "and when my friend bought a magazine and I was flipping through it, I was like, 'Holy cow, that's me!' It was one of those moments."

So has Mr Imboden fully adjusted to his dual life? "The biggest thing that worried me about getting into modelling was that I was going to have to wear some crazy things," he says. "It's a shock to the system when you look in the mirror and see someone else. But part of the cool thing about fashion is you can depict different things and be these different people."

THE KNOWLEDGE
TAILOR YOUR MIND

*The talks, tomes and topical websites to give
your brain the bespoke treatment*

Words by Mr Anthony Teasdale

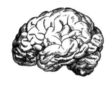

HAVING ALREADY PERUSED a few pages of this book, you'll
no doubt have your appearance down pat. But what about your
mind? In this informative guide, we provide eight pointers so that
your mind can remain as sharp as the cut of your suit.

I
GUNS, GERMS AND STEEL
By Professor Jared Diamond

Professor Diamond spent time in Papua New Guinea, studying the
traditional societies. One day, a local politician asked him: "If you
and I are as smart as each other, how come people from the West
have so much power?" His answer became the title of this tome,
in which he charts the history of Western man's rise, and looks at
why its privileged place came about due to its geographical good
fortune, communication links and proximity to food sources.

There are few more disheartening feelings than finding out that the "fact" that you've been wowing your friends and colleagues with for years is actually a myth. Happily, those with a thirst for real knowledge can check out the excellent Quora website. From the politics of Silicon Valley to the greatest steakhouse in Seattle, ask a question about any topic on Quora and soon enough it'll be answered, beating the illuminating *QI* quiz programme, hosted by Mr Stephen Fry, at its own game. And unlike other user-generated sites, Quora is noted for the civility of its contributors.

3

MINDFULNESS
By Professor Mark Williams and Dr Danny Penman

When you're in a position of responsibility either at home or work, having too many tasks to complete or even choices to make can be overwhelming and make you feel anxious and indecisive. Professor Williams and Dr Penman lay out a plan to combat this with the technique of mindfulness, which involves taking time out for just a few minutes a day to observe your own thoughts and feelings. Afterwards, you'll feel happier, sharper and able to see things in their true perspective. And you'll stop snapping at people.

4

THE MR PORTER PAPERBACK

Good news: you will have already discovered that MR PORTER provides a guide on how to dress, and more importantly, how to conduct oneself in modern society. Ideal for when you're facing those "Do I wear brown in town?" conundrums.

5
THE CIVIL WAR

Few documentary series can really be described as "great" – the Sir Laurence Olivier-narrated *The World at War* is one – but Mr Ken Burns' dissection of the American Civil War is perhaps the best of them all. More than 10 hours long, it tells the story of the war that set north against south, brother against brother and completely changed America from a loose conglomeration of states into a unified country – but at the cost of more than 700,000 lives. *The Civil War* took Mr Burns five years to make and garnered more than 40 awards – it's what DVD players were made for.

6
QUIET LEADERSHIP
By David Rock

As much a manifesto as a management book, *Quiet Leadership* intends to transform the way we think about management, basing its findings on scientific studies of the brain. With this knowledge, managers are able to work out how to make their teams happier, and consequently more productive. Which, if we have it right, should equate to more time for post-work cocktails – a most civilised way to reward collaboration.

7
DAN CARLIN'S HARDCORE HISTORY

Can't face the Kindle on your daily commute? Mr Dan Carlin's Hardcore History podcast is an excellent alternative, telling the story of the great events of the past in exhaustive detail. He brings passion and empathy to subjects including Genghis Khan's Mongol expansion and the collapse of the Roman Republic.

8

THREE TED TALKS THAT WILL MAKE
YOU LOOK AT THE WORLD ANEW

Lessons From Death Row
– Professor David R Dow

In this speech, Professor Dow illustrates why murderers seemingly all have the same biography – and how that can be used to prevent killings from happening in the future.

Where Good Ideas Come From
– Mr Steven Johnson

Mr Johnson's talk about what sparks creativity takes us from the coffee houses of 1700s London to the physics labs of 1950s America and the invention of GPS.

Underwater Astonishments
– Mr David Gallo

Humans have only explored 3% of the ocean, and Mr Gallo shows us what we're missing, including an astounding example of disguise by an extraordinary octopus.

16 MEN WHOSE DRESS
SENSE WE ADMIRE

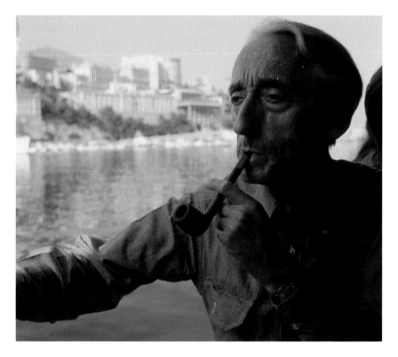

CAPTAIN JACQUES COUSTEAU

The world's most famous diver, who was a sort of marine-oriented, Gallic version of the BBC's Sir David Attenborough, combined elegant bearing with an enviable line in casual wear. We admire his habit of wearing a signature red beanie, but his button-down chambray shirts are genuinely inspirational.

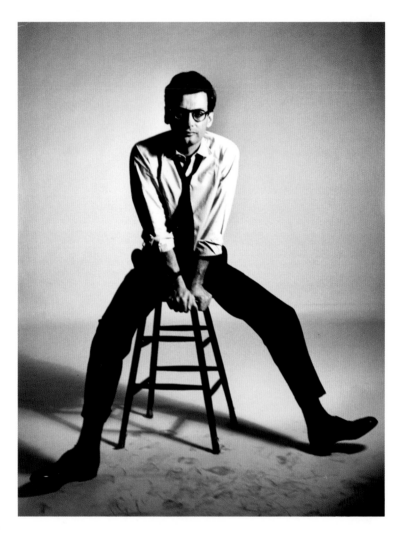

MR RICHARD AVEDON

One of the foremost fashion photographers of the second half of the 20th century, Mr Avedon enjoyed prodigious success under the mentorship of legendary art director Mr Alexey Brodovitch. As an expert in the image business, Mr Avedon knew that simplicity in dress is often the best option, particularly on formal occasions.

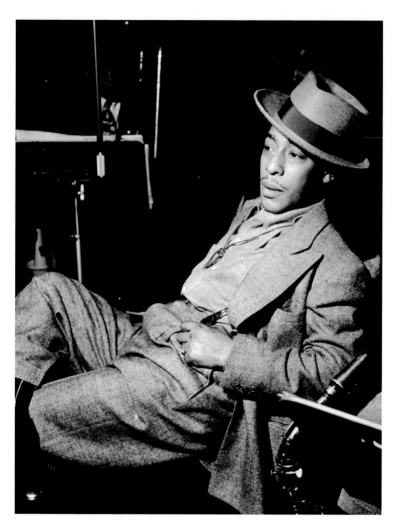

MR JOHNNY HODGES

This Bostonian saxophonist, like many jazz musicians, had a talent for dressing that rivalled his talent for playing. His look varied from the generously cut suits of the 1940s to more Bohemian styles in later decades, but he was never better dressed than when in this textured double-breasted suit. The way he wears it with a fedora is exemplary.

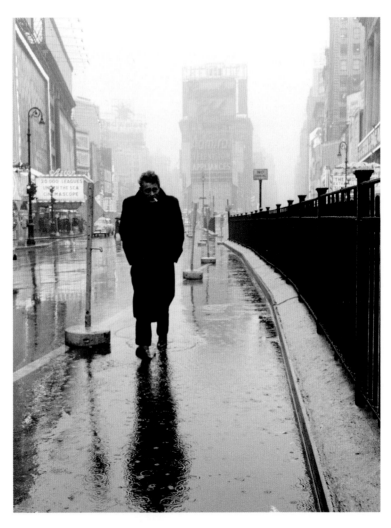

MR JAMES DEAN

Caught in a rain storm in Times Square, Mr Dean takes the opportunity to demonstrate that there's nothing stiff about overcoats, as long as you pick the right one. Buttoned up to the neck, and with the collar turned up against the weather, his double-breasted coat is practical, timeless and essential.

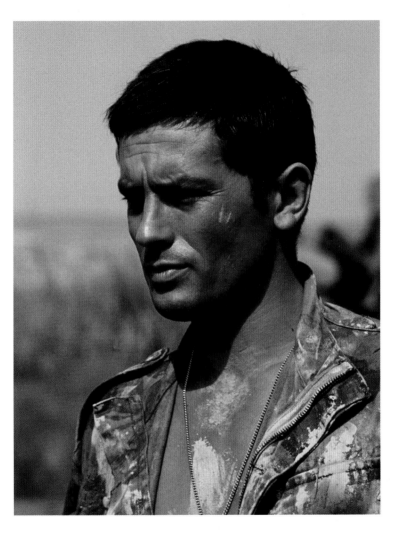

MR ALAIN DELON

The French-Swiss movie star may be known for wearing elegant
tailored clothes, not least his incomparable trench coat and trilby
outfit in the 1967 movie *Le Samouraï*, but in 1966's *Lost Command*
he demonstrated how to look just as stylish dressed down in army
fatigues. We're also impressed by the modern look of his haircut.

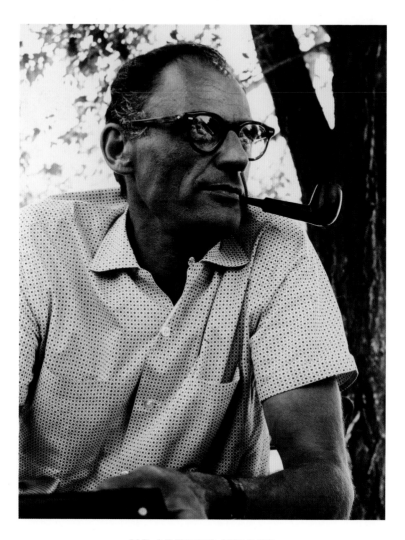

MR ARTHUR MILLER

The New York playwright may not have enjoyed matinée-idol looks but, encouragingly, he still married Ms Marilyn Monroe. Here he sports a printed shirt and a great pair of glasses while maintaining a literary intensity. We like to think it would still be a mixture potent enough to win the heart of a blonde bombshell.

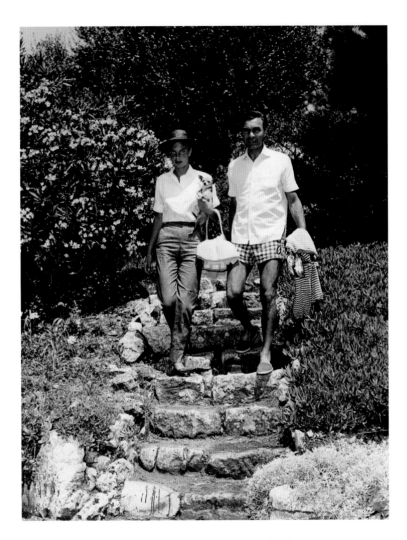

MR PORFIRIO RUBIROSA

As a faithful servant of Dominican dictator Rafael Trujillo, and the unfaithful husband to five wives, two of who were enormously rich American heiresses, Mr Rubirosa was no role model. However, with a lifestyle that included playing polo, racing at Le Mans, and driving Ferraris, he has something to teach us about good living.

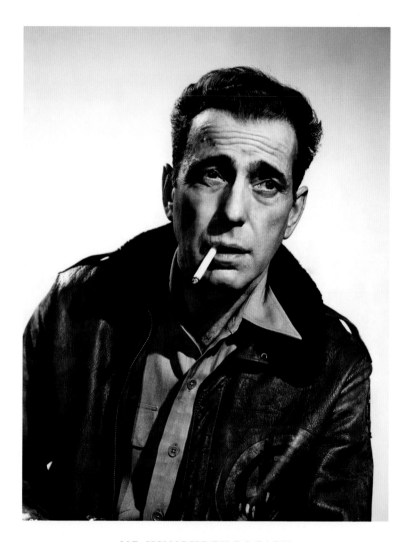

MR HUMPHREY BOGART

Mr Bogart, who is best known for the white tuxedo he wore in *Casablanca*, played an ex-serviceman in *Tokyo Joe*, who returns to the Japanese capital after WWII in search of his wife. The drapey suits he wears now look rather dated, but the way that he wears his relaxed-fitting flight jacket is anything but.

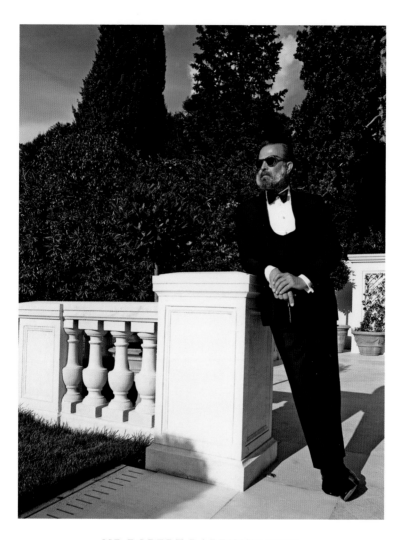

MR ROBERT RABENSTEINER

L'Uomo Vogue's fashion editor Mr Rabensteiner is renowned for mixing sophisticated soft tailoring with casual jeans, and introducing bold solid colours to his outfits. With these techniques he brings a modern attitude to fairly classic forms, something he deftly achieves with this three-piece midnight-blue dinner jacket.

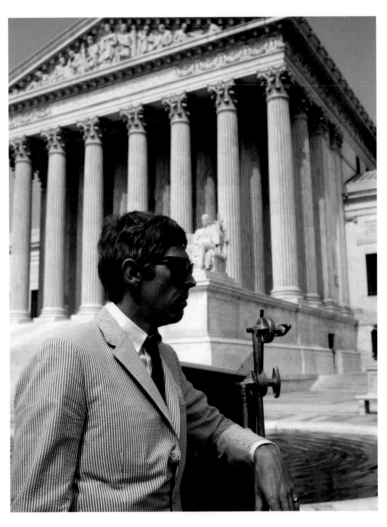

MR JAMES COBURN

The fact that this Hollywood tough guy had good taste is made clear by the cars he drove, which included a Ferrari Lusso and, famously, a 250 GT Spyder. It's hard to think of a better outfit in which to pilot a classic Italian sports car than a soft seersucker jacket, white shirt, slim tie and wraparound shades.

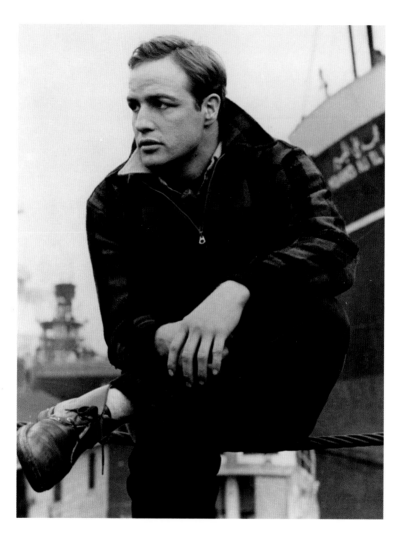

MR MARLON BRANDO

In the 1950s, a decade that saw him nominated five times for the Oscar for Best Actor, Mr Brando redefined what it meant to be a star. Mr Brando's casual style in his rugged workwear clothes in *On the Waterfront* has things to teach men even if the closest they'll get to the waterfront is stepping onto their yacht.

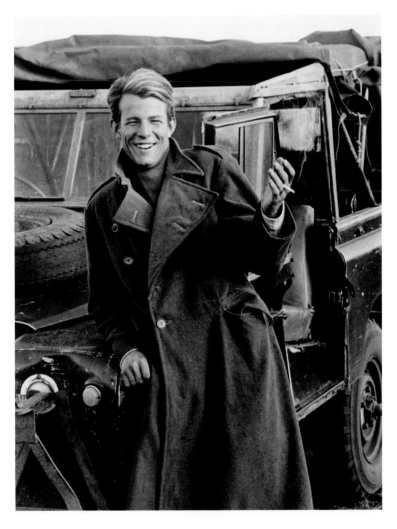

MR PETER BEARD

This highborn New Yorker, after being inspired by Ms Karen Blixen's *Out of Africa,* dedicated his career to recording his travels of the continent. His Bohemian style really clicks when in Africa – mixing Western clothes with native Kenyan dress. In this photo, we admire how his attitude takes all the formality out of a trench coat.

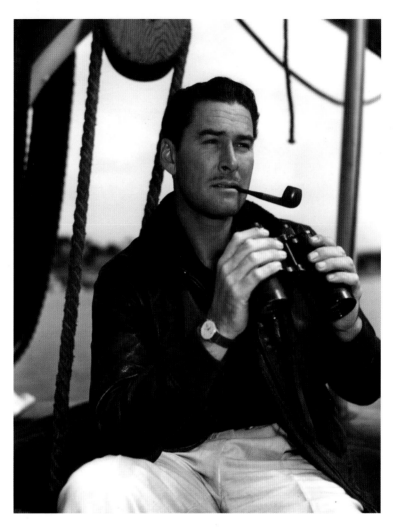

MR ERROL FLYNN

The Australian-born actor Mr Flynn, whose outfit here is only dated by the appearance of his pipe, was most often photographed in a jacket and tie. However, he looks far more at ease in this superb brown leather jacket, which reminds us that we've long promised ourselves a classic flight jacket.

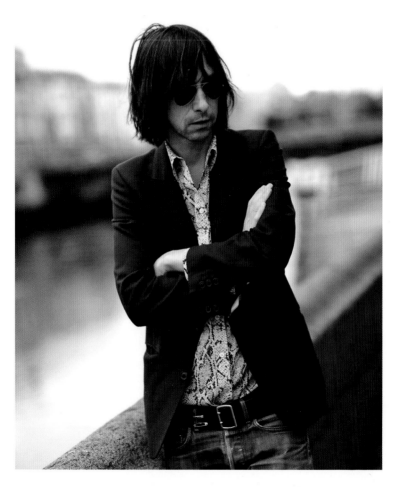

MR BOBBY GILLESPIE

The lead singer of British rock band Primal Scream has maintained an admirably consistent approach to style. Inspired by the classic rock look of The Velvet Underground, Mr Gillespie continues to wear slim jeans and Chelsea boots even now that he's celebrated his 50th birthday. He also wears a bold printed shirt with aplomb.

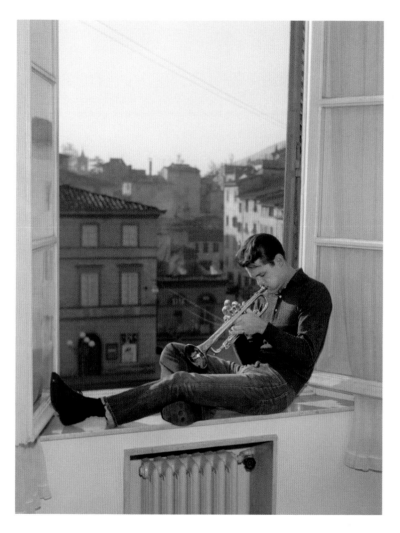

MR CHET BAKER

The US west coast jazz maestro, whose beautiful playing contrasted so strongly with his self-destructive lifestyle, wore simple clothes well. Back in 1961, playing his horn in Lucca, Italy, his long-sleeve shirt smartens up a pair of jeans. More than half a century later and this garment performs the exact same function.

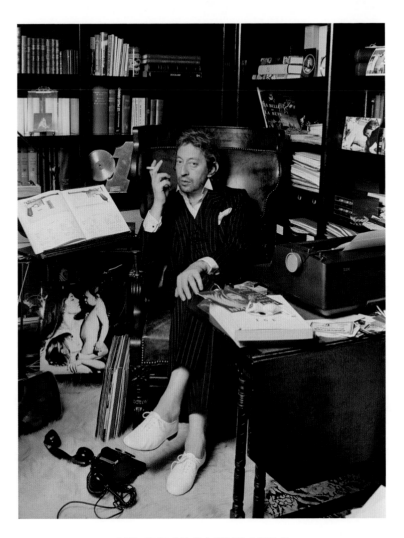

MR SERGE GAINSBOURG

This late French singer was a man who seemed to sum up the notion of roguish Gallic charm. He has set a fine example for men who want to make tailoring their own, as he demonstrates here in a three-piece pinstripe suit worn without a tie or socks, but with his favourite white Repetto dancing shoes.

THE REPORT

HOT DINNERS

MR PORTER *rounds up eight noteworthy restaurants from around the world*

Words by Mr John Lanchester

THE BROAD RULE of thumb with restaurants and food is the same as it is with all other areas of globalised life: you can get everything, everywhere, all the time. Produce is more internationalised than ever, and so are trends and cooking techniques – and as for the idea of keeping an idea secret, forget it. The bloggers and tweeters are across new developments as soon as they happen; no sooner has a chef put something on his menu for the first time than a customer has photographed it and uploaded it for the benefit of any chef in the world who wants to pinch, copy or imitate.

The important restaurant trend that has grown in response to this is to head in the opposite direction. It's about food that you precisely can't get anywhere else, or at any other moment: it's about unique experiences. Top chefs are now focused on locality and specificity. This cooking emphasises the sense of place. In the early noughties, the most influential restaurant in the world was generally agreed to be Mr Ferran Adrià's El Bulli on the Costa Brava, which was focused on technique and newness; these days its successor, Mr René Redzepi's Noma in Copenhagen, is all about locality, seasonality and sustainability. Here are eight places that exemplify the trend.

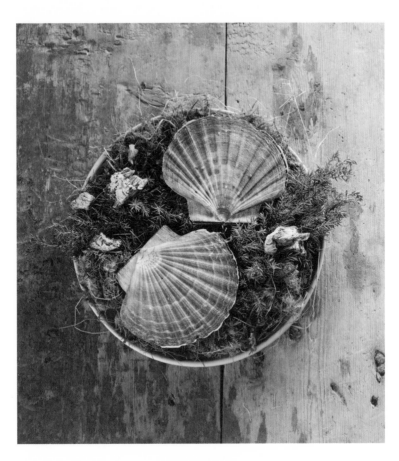

FÄVIKEN
Jäntland, Sweden

Anyone with the faintest interest in food knows that the Nordic region is where it's happening. There's a lot going on in the cities, especially Copenhagen and Stockholm, but one of the places that has generated considerable chatter is a lot further afield: the tiny, 12-cover Fäviken in the far north of Sweden. The chef, Mr Magnus Nilsson, is greatly admired by his peers for both his technical background – he worked for the great Mr Pascal Barbot at L'Astrance in Paris – and his down-home curing skills.

TIM HO WAN
Mongkok, Hong Kong

There may not be anywhere in the world with as great a concentration of people obsessed with food as there is in Hong Kong, and the city has a restaurant scene to match. With great options at every price point, why not go for one of the cheapest Michelin-starred restaurants in the world? Tim Ho Wan, a hole in the wall in Mongkok, serves dim sum that is as good as you can get anywhere, and if the queue looks too much – and there is always a queue – just waltz past and get something to take away.

MOMOFUKU SSÄM BAR
New York, US

The energetic, charismatic, original Korean-American chef Mr David Chang isn't so much a man as a movement, with a new idea or restaurant almost every month – let's open in Sydney! In Toronto! Let's start a magazine! Let's do a series for

PBS! You could try his 14-seat New York restaurant Ko, which everyone says is a) amazing and b) impossible to book. But to see what the fuss is about, go to Ssäm Bar, where Mr Chang's combination of superb palate, fine technique and love for both Asian and US influences combine to make a super-cool restaurant that continues to feel new.

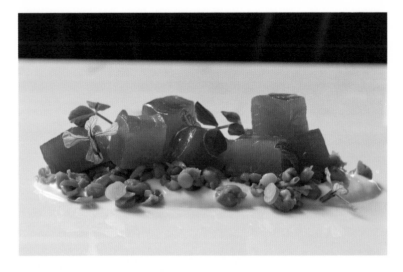

CUMULUS INC.
Melbourne, Australia

Australians love good food but dislike formality; the result is that nobody matches them for the combination of an informal vibe with ambitious cooking. Mr Andrew McConnell is a star of the Oz restaurant scene whose flagship venue, Cumulus Inc., is so relaxed in feeling that it's actually hard to believe how good it is, for anything from a breakfast cup of coffee and a croissant to an evening multi-course blow-out with wines to match. His cooking is innovative and bold but not in love with its own cleverness, and he takes a lot of trouble to make the vegetarian options as interesting as the others.

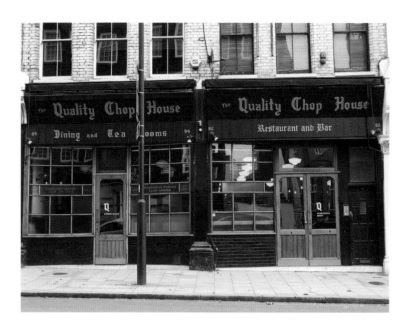

THE QUALITY CHOP HOUSE
London, UK

One of the great restaurant interiors in London, preserved intact from the 1869 design of Mr Rowland Plumbe, with the intention of being (as the window etching says) a "Progressive Working Class Caterer". One of the working-class heroes who reopened the Chop House in 2012 is the son of wine and food critic legends Ms Jancis Robinson and Mr Nick Lander, and it shows: the restaurant and bar are assured, professional, and offer good grazing and drinking options including the sublime four-course dinner.

MUGARITZ
San Sebastián, Spain

San Sebastián is the world's culinary capital, and its best young chef, Mr Andoni Luis Aduriz, is the leader of his generation of chefs in Spain. To see what the fuss is about, you must visit his restaurant Mugaritz – the word meaning "border oak" – a few miles outside the city. (Take a cab, you'll never find it on your own.) His food is both disorienting and comforting, and ranges from fossilised salsify and clay-covered potatoes to the best eggy bread you'll ever taste. For cooking at this level, ie the world, it's also sensational value.

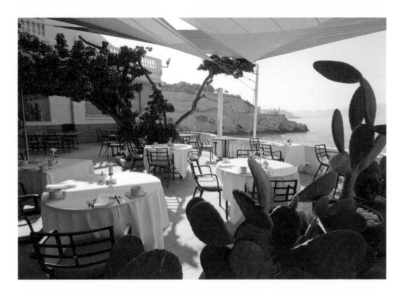

LE PETIT NICE
Marseille, France

So much of the Mediterranean coast is an architectural and culinary disaster zone that it can feel impossible to find a place combining the setting, the scenery, the food and the service. Don't give up: Le Petit Nice, on the Corniche in Marseille, is that place. Now run by the third generation of the Passédat family – the head chef is Mr Gérald Passédat – the restaurant focuses on the exquisite local seafood, tweaked by influences from further afield. Its lightness fits the location, with a view out over the bay that you won't want to leave, or forget.

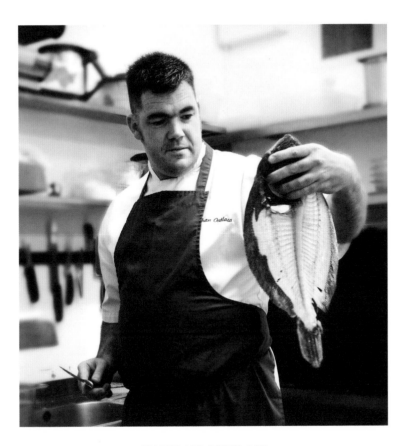

NATHAN OUTLAW
Cornwall, UK

I don't think there's a chef anywhere in the world with a better name than Mr Nathan Outlaw, whose eponymous seafood restaurant is in the Cornish village of Rock. His cooking is fancy enough to have won two Michelin stars, but the great thing about it is that it doesn't feel fancy at all: simple and direct, it focuses on getting the most flavour out of incredible produce. The tasting menu (the only kind available) is beautifully thought through, with a lovely balance between the individual high spots and the overall shape of the meal.

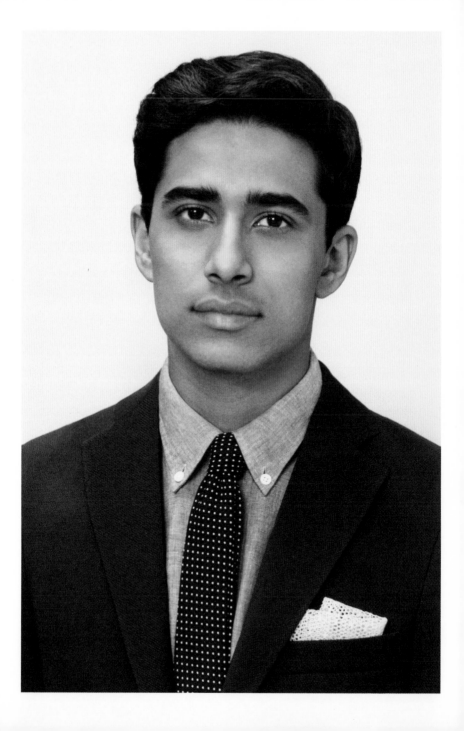

MR SURAJ SHARMA

The charming Life of Pi *actor on meditation,*
diets, and why he may never act again

Words by Mr Alex Godfrey

MANY ACTORS talk of films being life-changing experiences.
With *Life of Pi*, Mr Suraj Sharma has had his entire existence
flipped, transformed, turned upside down and inside out. Before
he was cast at the age of 17, he'd never acted; he couldn't swim;
he'd never left India. He grew up in suburban South Delhi, the
son of an economist mother and a software engineer father.
He was at school, half-heartedly training to be an economist
when his younger brother asked him to accompany him to the
Life of Pi auditions, as he didn't want to go on his own. The
casting director told him he might as well try out too. Now he
finds himself in a position of global acclaim and stardom, his
life a constant stream of premieres, promotions and parties. Not
that you'd know it. He's a wonderfully relaxed, playful model
at our shoot, humble and charming, with no sign of the eternal
jet lag he's enduring. Cast from 3,000 hopefuls, it's clear what
Mr Ang Lee saw in him – his gentle, lovely spirit matches that of
the film. And although he says he may never act again, whatever he
does do with his life it's sure to be something great.

Do you think it worked in your favour that you weren't an actor?
Yeah. Ang said the fact that I wasn't trained allowed him to mould me into whatever he wanted. So I was trying to find my way out as the story moved along. I was acting; my character was trying to survive. But we were both going into the unknown, trying to figure out what needed to be done.

I read on the second audition you did with Mr Lee that you started crying. What happened?
He talked to me in a certain way, put me in a state of mind. You take him seriously whenever he speaks. He's very soft-spoken so you're trying to listen even harder, you end up concentrating a lot. And he's trying to make you understand that you basically need to find the same emotion as the character. You don't need to be in the same spot, but being in that emotional state, inside you are in the same spot, in some senses. So that's what he did. And it was a long scene. The emotion built up and up and up to the point where crying seemed appropriate.

I read that in order to look emaciated in the film, you were on a tuna and lettuce diet for three months. Did you pig out when you got off it?
I couldn't. My stomach shrank. When I was 14 I could eat a 14" pizza and then another half pizza. Now I can't even eat half. My stomach's grown since the day the diet finally ended, but it's a very slow pace. The day I finished, I tried pigging out – that was the idea. I had a lot of dumplings, fattening food, but I couldn't handle much. Before the diet I used to have 40 dumplings every day. That time I could only handle 11.

So the film's made you healthier.
Most definitely. Stronger, healthier. I can swim now and control my breathing. I have a deeper understanding of how my body and mind work together.

I know you spent a lot of time meditating with Mr Lee. What did that involve, and how did it benefit you?

Lots of focusing and relaxing our bodies and minds. You enter your cave and understand yourself better, you can fill yourself with light. By the end of it all you're in a perpetual state of meditation: things happen around you, not to you. On set I was being beaten up by everything but I was completely OK with it, as if I was sitting with a whirlwind around me. Just sitting there, and it's cool.

I wonder if Mr Lee does that on other films, or if it was specific to this one because of your character's isolation.

I've met a couple of actors he's worked with and they gave me the sense that he goes deeper than what is considered normal. He told me once that his understanding of his actors, and theirs of him, is far deeper than what he can have with anybody else. Because he really allows you to come inside his mind. You see what he's trying to project and you become part of that picture.

He was giving you acting coaching too – by the time it came to shooting were you completely confident about it?

No, I didn't know if I could act yet. I feel as if Ang directed me right. I don't know who else can direct me right. That's my fear. We'll see.

This must have been an intense film to make, and in terms of acting you were on your own a lot. Did you have vivid dreams while you were making it?

I did. It was disturbing. There was a phase which I've termed the dark age. For me. For a month Ang told everybody not to talk to me, so I'd have complete isolation. I was just meditating on my own or going through this super-crazy work-out. I was hungry, thirsty, extremely tired, awake. And my dreams would be very dark. I would wake up very disturbed. I would wake up feeling, Jesus Christ... I felt as if there was a problem with me. There was a dream about an ocean and a boat going in, the water was going down into an abyss, it was all around me. It really messed me up. It was as weird as hell. I can't get that image out of my head.

Do you get treated differently at home now?
Yes. I don't like it. I appreciate that people appreciate your work; it's nice to know they like it. But I don't like attention. At all.

You're in the wrong industry.
I know. It's one thing I'm just weirded out by. I can't deal with it, I'm extremely awkward. People coming up to me, it bothers me.

Is that one of the things that would put you off acting again?
Yeah. That is *the* thing. That is it. The idea of fame or recognition, I don't want that at all. I love acting because you discover billions of things about yourself, you feel so free, like a bird, but suddenly that bird gets caged. Because you're always hiding, in that sense.

If you were cast in another film but it meant spending three months in a wave tank again...
I'd do it. Totally do it. I would go through all that again, any day. Oh my God. It was all horribly amazing.

SALONE DEL MOBILE

MR PORTER meets six leading designers from the Milan furniture
fair who are shaping the future of Italian design

Words by Mr Nick Vinson

MILAN'S Salone del Mobile is by far the biggest furniture fair in the world. More than 324,000 visitors flock to Milan each April to see the new launches from leading furniture brands. The fair is held in the Mr Massimiliano Fuksas-designed fairgrounds in Rho, where 2,500 exhibitors fill the exhibition space, while 400 others show in the city itself. The fair's protagonists are the world-class architects who, when not busy building museums, hotels or retail cathedrals, put their talents into product design. We talked to six of these clever chaps about Italian design and what the fair means to them.

MR MARIO BELLINI
Architect and designer

Mr Mario Bellini graduated from the Politecnico di Milano in 1959 and was already renowned as both an architect and designer as early as 1963. Winner of no less than eight Compasso d'Oro, the "Oscars" of the design world, he also boasts 25 works in the prestigious permanent design collection of MoMA in New York. Mr Bellini's more recent projects include renovating the Pinacoteca di Brera in Milan and designing the Department of Islamic Art in the Louvre.

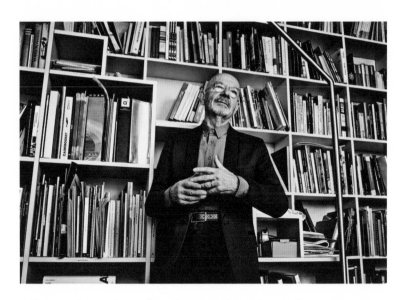

What is it that makes Italian design and "made in Italy" so unique?
It was determined by the way it built itself up after WWII. Italy was devastated; the small courageous industries immediately started to think how to rebuild and survive. We did not have big industries like in the US or Germany, so because of this, it was spontaneous. These entrepreneurs felt free to follow new ideas, experiment and take risks. We had various young architects who did not have too much to perform with architecture so they turned to design, then part of the same field.

Why do you think Milan is a focus of both design and fashion?
Designers from all over the world come to work with small- and medium-sized companies to produce what we call Italian design. During the early 1970s young fashion designers started coming out like flowers in Milan; little by little it became strong. All around us we have great handcraft. It has something special; fashion, furniture or design, there is a spirit and a dynamic. There is the critical mass effect, so now you need to be here.

Italian design is known the world over. Why do you think that is?
More and more it's performed by designers from all over the world but it's still Italian, because they need B&B Italia, Cassina, Edra to produce it.

Why do architecture, design and fashion cross over so much?
We are in physical contact with our clothing and furniture. Fashion is fashion, architecture is architecture, but they have common roots that always refer to the human body and habitation. That is the relationship.

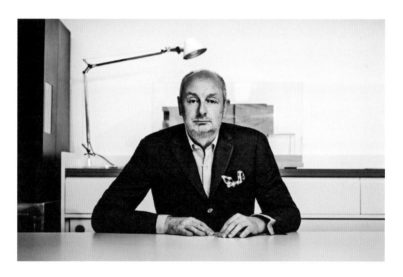

MR PIERO LISSONI
Architect and designer

Lissoni Associati was founded in Milan in 1986, and today a team of 60 designs everything from hotels and showrooms to furniture and lighting. Perhaps unique to Mr Piero Lissoni is the addition of art direction, corporate identity, advertising, graphic design and packaging design, making him a one-stop shop for creative competence with a clean, contemporary feel.

What is it that makes Italian design and "made in Italy" so unique?
It's so easy; it's the factories and the boundaries. You have to think handcraft culture. It does not matter if you use robots or hands; Italy is the perfect place to be.

Why do you think Milan is a focus of both design and fashion?
Everything is connected and Milan is in the middle; it's possible to combine things together. And it's a special culture of connection and contamination – somebody very good at making shoes can help someone who can make chairs. It's a crossover place.

Italian design is known the world over. Why do you think that is?
It's not done by the Italians. Design is a system. We are not chauvinists. It's an incredible mishmash of cultures.

Why do architecture, design and fashion cross over so much?
Now to be good in fashion you have to sell your products in a particular space. I like it when you are in the middle of the stage. Architecture is a combination and a link with inside and outside. There is a link with different processes.

MR MATTEO THUN
Architect and designer

Mr Matteo Thun founded Sottsass Associati with the legendary Ettore Sottsass in 1980 before setting up his own office in Milan. Today Matteo Thun & Partners has a team of more than 50 working internationally on architectural, interior and product design projects. Mr Thun's architectural work focuses on sustainability and environment, illustrated in the Hugo Boss Business Unit in Coldrerio, Switzerland, and concept store in New York. The Vigilius Mountain Resort and Terme Merano, both in South Tyrol, make him the go-to man for resorts that fit seamlessly into exquisite natural settings.

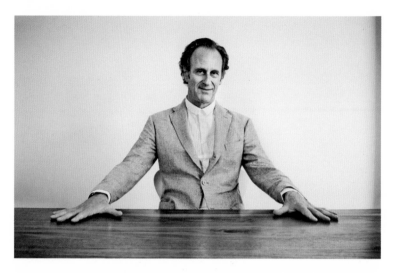

What is it that makes Italian design and "made in Italy" so unique?
The tradition, the history, food, architecture, art and the art of life. After all we have the worst performance of democracy, yet the art of life survives.

Why do you think Milan is a focus of both design and fashion?
Foreigners believe so, and all the 60 or so who work in my office think they are in the centre. Surprisingly the Milan nightlife is great for the youngsters.

Italian design is known the world over. Why do you think that is?
It's not about Italian design, it's about a holistic approach working in architecture, interiors, light design and styling. This is called the Milan school; it's anti-academic, as normally you learn one but not all together.

Why do architecture, design and fashion cross over so much?
This city gives you the opportunity to be in a big family, and friendship between parties gives a crossover of information. Milan is a small town; we meet for dinner, for parties, and we exchange.

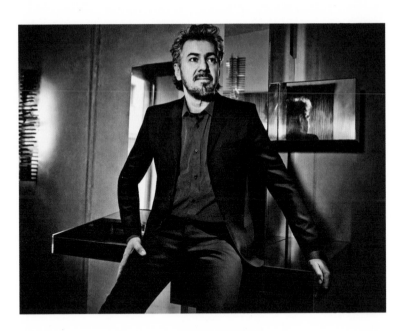

MR VINCENZO DE COTIIS
Architect and artist

Mr Vincenzo de Cotiis creates architecture for hotels, homes and stores and designs for Rossana, Ceccotti Collezioni and Busnelli. He more often than not reappropriates found materials and crafts them into new volumes and shapes. If you know where to look, Milan is full of Mr de Cotiis' treasures, such as the Straf hotel, Sportmax and Excelsior stores, and his own Galleria De Cotiis of limited-edition furniture.

What is it that makes Italian design and "made in Italy" so unique?
In my opinion it's the background and, first and foremost, the artisanal experience, combined with technology.

Why do you think Milan is a focus of both design and fashion?
It is the capital of Italian creativity and the city where international culture mixes.

Italian design is known the world over. Why do you think that is?
Because there is a big capacity to realise and produce, and a grand
professionalism and a history of Italian design. This makes up the
furniture fair.

Why do architecture, design and fashion cross over so much?
I think that it's a cultural phenomenon, above all design and
fashion. Architecture is a culture; design and fashion absorb the
various international cultures and become eclectic.

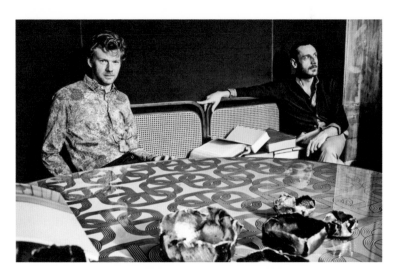

MESSRS EMILIANO SALCI & BRITT MORAN
Interior designers

Established in 2003 by Messrs Emiliano Salci and Britt Moran,
Dimore Studio assembles eras past and present, mixing vintage
and contemporary in a highly stylised way. Projects of note include
rooms, suites and the Caruso bar/restaurant at the Grand Hotel et
de Milan, Caffè Burlot in Paris and The Pump Room in Chicago.
In 2012 Dimore Studio worked with Mr Tomas Maier of Bottega
Veneta for the presentation of the brand's home collection.

What is it that makes Italian design and "made in Italy" so unique?
Perhaps what makes it so unique is the craftsmanship in Italy
and everything that is created here. Italians have an ability to see
things, the details. We have a small group of artisans we use that
gives us the handcrafted look we are after.

Why do you think Milan is a focus of both design and fashion?
Because among the small and large workshops miracles and
dreams are produced. Then there is the fact that Milan is closer to
the rest of Europe.

Italian design is known the world over. Why do you think that is?
Historically Italian designers had amazing taste. The timeless
pieces, known all over the world, look good in all types of spaces.
Today Italians like to experiment and take risks, both with ideas
and economically, a total risk. Italians are a bit childish, not totally
rational, very colourful, exhibitionists and open to collaborations
with foreigners.

Why do architecture, design and fashion cross over so much?
In today's work everything is related, especially with colour
and fabric. Information is very immediate; we are all much
better informed.

MR JAMES MCNEILL WHISTLER

The 19th century's most quick-witted artist,
who caused a stir with what he said, painted and wore

Words by Mr Colin McDowell

MR JAMES MCNEILL WHISTLER could never be called a quiet American. Even today when there are thousands of Americans living in London he would stand out. In the last years of the 19th century he was as well-known in London's social circles as Mr Beau Brummel had been 100 years earlier. And like the legendary dandy, Mr Whistler was a dude, a wit and a poseur. He was also one of the most controversial men of his time.

Born in Massachusetts in 1834, Mr Whistler had itchy feet and was ready to take on the world from an early age. He loved Europe and even spent a year in St Petersburg as a young man. He studied at West Point, America's top army training college, where he was eventually sacked because even in his youth he was a contrarian. Always ready to argue with anyone over anything – a propensity that was to get him into trouble throughout his life – he made no attempt to fit in or go with the crowd. But for those who found him insufferable there were many more who found his company delightful and his challenging attitudes endlessly stimulating.

Mr Whistler was a social entertainer, always sharply critical and ready with a witty comment. He was once entertaining a group of London's intellectuals and after an especially witty comment, the poet Mr Oscar Wilde, who was a friend, said, "I wish I had said that, James". The reply came as quick as a flash: "You will, Oscar, you will." It's little wonder that when it came to his paintings, Mr Whistler signed them with a butterfly with a long stinger tail. It showed that he knew what he was made of – gentle, even fragile delicacy but with a sharp sting in the tail for those who crossed him or stood in the way of his boundless ambition. But while he may have had many of the characteristics of a street-fighting bruiser, his paintings were as understated as any great painters.

Mr Whistler was a great painter, and is recognised as such, although fashion has changed and he is now no longer at the forefront. At the time of his best work, his strange approach to naming them brought him criticism for being pretentious. He called them by musical names, such as nocturnes or harmonies. The most famous of all his work was the portrait of his mother, which he called "Arrangement in Grey and Black". It became one of the most famous paintings of the time and was bought by the Musée D'Orsay in Paris, where it still holds pride of place.

A man with such a single-minded attitude could be expected to have an original approach to his appearance, and Mr Whistler certainly did. There was nothing about him that was not contrived. Everything was for effect. By no means conventionally handsome, and slight of figure, he had a dominating presence nevertheless. It was all about swagger and style. From his ringlets, usually half hidden under a floppy velvet cap reminiscent of Rembrant, to his long silver-topped cane without which he was rarely seen, this little man somehow contrived to have a large presence. His monocle glinting with malice, his dandy clothes – almost always black and tight, to show off his slight figure – and his curling moustache made him stand out from the crowd. People noticed him even before he opened his mouth and let the outrageous comments flow.

And it was this that got him into trouble. Nothing if not arrogant, he was incensed when Mr John Ruskin, the man considered the greatest art critic in Victorian England, wrote of one of Mr Whistler's "Nocturne" paintings, "I have heard much of cockney

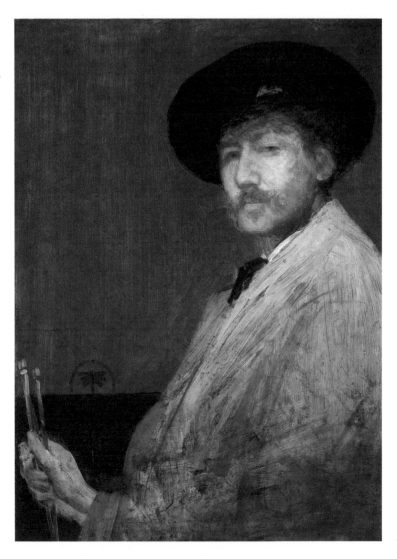

"Arrangement in Gray: Portrait of the Painter"
by Mr James McNeill Whistler, circa 1872

impudence before now; but never expected to hear a coxcomb ask two hundred guineas [a huge amount at that time] for flinging a pot of paint in the public's face." It was a red rag to a bull for Mr Whistler, who responded by suing Mr Ruskin for libel. The trial was a society occasion with crowds waiting for entrance to the court. After all, a public scrap between a major art critic and one of society's sharpest wits could not fail to be entertaining. And it was. Choosing his words to convey the greatest contempt for the painting in question, Mr Ruskin's lawyer asked Mr Whistler, "How long did it take you to knock it off?" When Mr Whistler replied that it had taken two days, the lawyer said, "The labour of two days? Is that for which you ask 200 guineas?" Mr Whistler rose to the occasion. "No. I ask it for the knowledge I have gained in the work of a lifetime." The public gallery stood up and cheered him. He won the day. But this time the sting in the tail was aimed at him. While he won his case, the libel damages, rather than thousands, were in fact exactly one farthing. His exuberance never recovered from the blow to his self-esteem and his standing in public opinion.

WOMEN OF NOTE
MS RITA ORA

*The stunning British pop star on the
five tracks that move her the most*

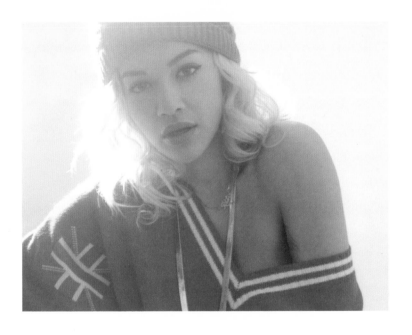

"Don't Speak"
NO DOUBT

"Gwen Stefani is a role model of mine and this is the song that got
me hooked on the band. She's so confident and the guys are so cool.
What's not to like?"

"No Ordinary Love"
SADE

"She's my dad's favourite singer so he would play her in our house all the time when I was younger. I love her voice and passion – and the video's amazing too!"

"I Will Wait"
MUMFORD & SONS

"I love the way they use their words in such a simple way. It just clicks and they really make you feel a part of it – it's amazing."

"Party and Bullshit"
THE NOTORIOUS B.I.G.

"I grew up in West London so hip-hop was a big influence for me. This was without doubt one of my favourite tunes."

"Crazy in Love"
BEYONCÉ

"This was such an anthem. I love powerful women and Beyoncé represents that as well as anyone."

THE REPORT

LE CORBUSIER

We look at the life and style of modernism's master architect

Words by Ms Alice Rawsthorn,
design critic, *International Herald Tribune*

ON LE CORBUSIER'S first visit to New York, to open an exhibition of his architecture at the Museum of Modern Art in October 1935, he was so enthralled by the skyscrapers – by the Empire State Building especially – that he told a friend: "I wanted to lie down on my back there on the sidewalk, and gaze towards the top forever."

Then in his late forties, Le Corbusier was in the vanguard of the "rads versus trads" battle in design: idolised by fellow radicals, and loathed by conservative "trads". Nearly 50 years after his death, MoMA honoured him with another, far larger exhibition in 2013, which helped seal his reputation as the most influential architect of the modern age.

Just as contemporary art would not be the same without Mr Marcel Duchamp, literature without Mr James Joyce, or fashion without Mr Yves Saint Laurent, our built environment – from houses and schools to towns and cities – would be very different if not for Le Corbusier. But why?

Like most other visionaries who revolutionised their fields, Le Corbusier was blessed not only with exceptional talent, but great timing. He began his career in the early 1900s when the availability of electricity, telephones, aeroplanes and cars was transforming people's lives. Every aspect of society needed to be rethought, including architecture, a challenge that Le Corbusier relished. "The time is ripe for construction," he wrote, "not foolery."

His first design project was himself. Born Charles-Édouard Jeanneret-Gris in 1887 in La Chaux-de-Fonds, a sleepy Swiss watchmaking town, he began his career there before moving to Paris in 1917. He promptly rechristened himself "Le Corbusier" by adopting his maternal grandfather's surname, and took to wearing the horn-rimmed glasses that became his trademark. Equally adept at moulding perceptions of his work, he tinkered with photographs of his buildings (often using his glasses as props) and wrote so prolifically that other architects were as familiar with his thinking as his appearance. His mediagenic successors, from Mr Rem Koolhaas to Ms Zaha Hadid, have since adopted similar strategies to cultivate equally distinctive identities.

But Le Corbusier's true legacy is his architecture. During the 1920s, he pioneered the "machine aesthetic", or International Style, by applying newly developed materials and construction techniques, often discovered in other fields, such as the automotive and aerospace industries, to produce geometric, white-walled structures such as the elegant Villa Savoye and his other "purist villas" in and around Paris.

From the late 1930s onwards he began combining concrete with natural materials such as wood and stone to create a robust organic style of architecture dubbed "brutalism". These experiments culminated in post-war gems such as the Notre Dame du Haut chapel in Ronchamp in eastern France and Chandigarh, the "City Beautiful" that he designed in northern India, whose majestic concrete buildings were surrounded by greenery.

In the machine aesthetic and brutalism, Le Corbusier defined the dominant architectural styles of the 20th century. Other architects attempted them too, but rarely with such aplomb. Technocratic though he was, Le Corbusier also understood the sensual aspects of architecture, doubtless because he was an accomplished painter. He imbued his buildings with a cinematic quality by orchestrating

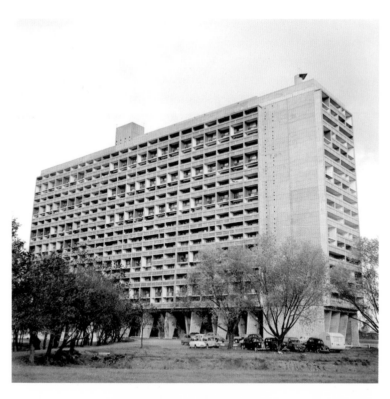

L'Unité d'Habitation, Marseille, 1952

the experience of being there so skilfully that anyone encountering them will see something seductive wherever they look.

Even so, Le Corbusier has proved as contentious since his death as he was during his life, not least by being blamed for the dreary state of post-war architecture. How can he be held responsible for the design crimes of his imitators, when his work was so inspiring?

Take his mass housing project, L'Unité d'Habitation in Marseille, whose subtly sculpted concrete is enlivened by light, colour, texture and greenery, just like Chandigarh. As the German architect Mr Walter Gropius said at the opening party: "Any architect who does not find this building beautiful had better lay down his pencil."

Le Corbusier's personal style was almost as distinctive as his architecture: round, thick-rimmed glasses and double-breasted jackets with broad lapels, usually worn with a pocket square and bow tie, made up his signature look and set the precedent for the "architect" style of dressing. He was not afraid to wear an immaculate three-piece suit while drawing, but was equally adept at dressing down in flannel trousers and a patterned blazer. Le Corbusier's life was a stylish one, and there was even something oddly elegant about his death: aged 77, and defying his doctor's orders, Le Corbusier went for a swim in the Mediterranean sea near Monaco and never returned.

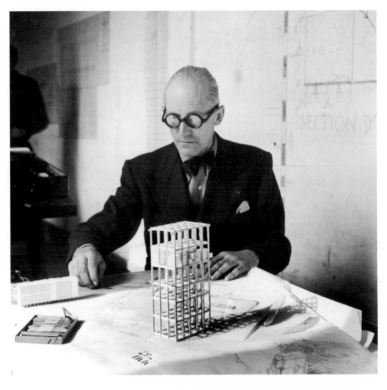

A portrait of Le Corbusier as he looks at architectural plans and a building model in his offices, Paris, May 1946

THE KNACK
(AND HOW TO GET IT)

Experts offer practical advice
on a variety of life's more unexpected,
as well as conventional, conundrums

HOW TO BE A MUSIC BUFF

By Mr Tim Jonze, music editor at guardian.co.uk

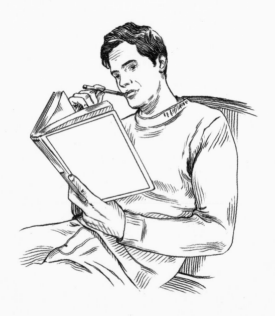

BEING A MUSIC BUFF may look easy to the observer – after all, what could be challenging about going to gigs and spinning the odd record? Pah! These people know little of the blood, sweat and learning of rare B-sides that goes into being a serious musical connoisseur. It feels like a full-time job to reach the peaks of music fandom, involving hours of research, relentless one-upmanship and a delicate relationship with your own sanity. But then, nobody ever said being a music fan was supposed to be fun, right?

1
IDENTIFY YOUR GENRES

Knowing your free jazz from your folktronica might seem as if it will take forever, but you only really need to grasp the basics to get by. Listen to key tracks online and look out for each genre's trademark sounds. A punishing and relentless beat? That'll be techno. A bass wobble so powerful that it sets your bowels in motion? Most likely dubstep. A hairy man shouting over riffs in a way not entirely acquainted with the concept of melody? That, my friend, will be heavy metal.

2
CHOOSE A SPECIALIST AREA

It's the norm for music aficionados to say they like "a bit of everything", adopting the casual air of someone equally at home at a country-rock convention as they are at a sweatbox dancehall rave in Kingston. In reality, though, we all need to specialise, so have no shame in being the authority on West Coast psychedelic rock circa 1968 if that's what floats your boat – just make sure you know the name of every single by The Electric Prunes. And release date. And catalogue number.

3
DRESS THE PART

Feeling at home in your musical genre, especially at gigs, often involves a degree of sartorial adjustment. Skinny jeans are still *de rigueur* at indie gigs, for example, as are quiffs. Anything vaguely folky or pastoral is best enjoyed with a plaid shirt and a fulsome beard. If you find yourself in a Barbour jacket and wellies while carrying a banjo then you have inadvertently become a Mumford & Sons fan and need to take a long hard look in the mirror.

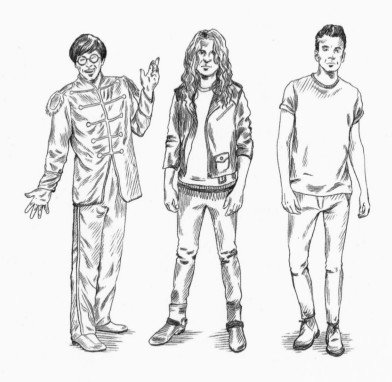

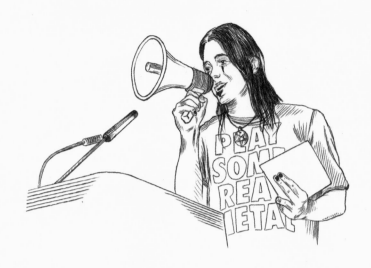

4
GET INVOLVED

Music fandom isn't about watching from the sidelines. DIY or DIE is the mantra, so try contributing to the scene you love the most. Start up a blog or put on a few live gigs at your local venue. Better still, have a go at releasing records yourself – surprisingly fun if writing limited-edition numbers on 500 pieces of cardboard is your idea of a great Saturday night in.

5
KNOW THE LINGO

Specialist music forums can be intimidating jungles of acronyms (BPM! LFO!) and alien terms. At first you may feel the need to feed large chunks into Google Translate, but you must persevere, for no music buff wants to be heard saying: "You know, that wibbly synth bit in the middle." Learn about low-end frequencies at *dubstepforum.com*, whereas Pitchfork is the place for chillwave and cloud rap.

BE OPINIONATED

This is where you graduate from rookie to bona fide annoying know-it-all. A good way to start throwing around your attention-grabbing, unasked-for opinions is by dismantling sacred cows. Call Prince overrated or try to argue that Maroon 5 are superior songsmiths to The Beach Boys. Actually, no, don't do that one.

SOME COMMON MISTAKES

BEING TOO SLOW

There's no point telling people about the new Frank Ocean album when everyone else has already moved on to raving over Miguel. As with making wisecracks on Twitter, being first is everything in this game.

NOT BEING OBSCURE ENOUGH

If music buffery is your world then consider obscurity your currency. Nobody will be impressed by your suggestion to go seek out *Abbey Road*. A Transylvanian trip-hop collective that only formed last Wednesday, however…

ADMITTING THAT YOU'RE BLAGGING IT

Have you just rhapsodised about Justin Timberlake's excellent hip-hop productions only to be met with sniggers and "You mean Timbaland, right?" You could, of course, admit that you're clueless. Then again you could just shrug and say: "Maybe you've just never heard those tracks…" before walking away, very quickly.

HOW TO WASH A CAR LIKE A PRO

By Mr Walter Gray, foreman at Lellers Car Valeting Service

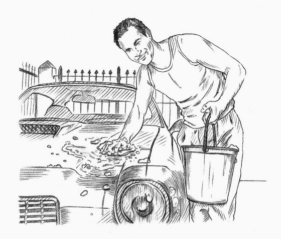

FOUNDED IN 1986 in Hertfordshire, England, Lellers has become the pre-eminent name in British car valeting. The company, which operates two sites in central London, as well as one in Hertfordshire, cleans cars for companies including Ferrari, Jaguar, Aston Martin and Lamborghini, as well as visiting leading London hotels and private customers all over England. And so, Mr Walter Gray is well placed to advise on that most masculine of activities – washing cars. If the full wash that he recommends sounds exhausting then bear in mind his useful tip: "If you are pushed for time just clean the wheels, windows and dashboard. As long as these are taken care of your car will feel clean."

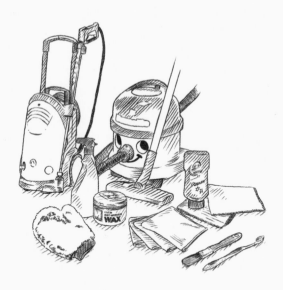

1
YOU'LL NEED

A jet washer, wheel-cleaning fluid, a toothbrush to clean the wheels, a small paintbrush to dust around the switching, a vacuum cleaner, a wash mitt, a cloth with which to clean the windows, auto wax for the bodywork and windows, vinyl polish for the tyres and for black bumpers, and microfibre cloths to clean and dry the car.

2
THE MUD

Use a jet wash to spray all the mud and debris off the bodywork, especially inside the wheel arches. A lot of people don't clean inside the wheel arches, but that's where rust can start because caked mud stays moist, and it can even affect the way a car handles. We use tar and glue remover to clean the paint around the bottom of the car; leave it on for 10 minutes before wiping it off.

3
THE WHEELS

Spray the wheel cleaner onto the alloys before using the jet washer to clean them. Then move the car forward so the wheels turn 180 degrees, and repeat. Use a toothbrush to clean inside the grooves. We finish the tyres with a vinyl polish.

4
THE INTERIOR

Open all the doors and the boot. Starting on one side of the car, and then working around it, clean all the shuts and then vacuum the interior, including the boot. Use a small paintbrush to remove the dust that gathers around the switches. Clean the dashboard with a microfibre cloth.

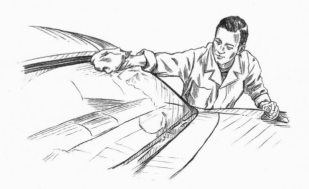

5
THE WINDOWS

I start with the driver's window, and clean the inside and then the outside. You have to do them together otherwise you can't see which side of the glass the marks are on. Use a special window cloth, and if there are watermarks polish the glass with car polish.

6

THE BODYWORK

Start on the bonnet, and work around the car one panel at a time. If it's a hot day, or a big car, then clean one half of the car and dry it before starting on the other half. This will prevent water drying on the bodywork and creating streaks. Dry the bodywork with a microfibre cloth soaked in water mixed with car polish, which helps the water to run off. Apply a layer of polish, which protects the paint, between once a month and every six weeks.

SOME COMMON MISTAKES

GATHERING DUST

Using polish on the dashboard will leave a residue that will attract dust and fluff.

STREAKING

Failing to dry the windows after you've washed them will result in streaks when the water evaporates.

SCRATCHING THE PAINT

Using a sponge on the bodywork before you've used a high-pressure hose to remove all mud and debris will cause grit to get caught under the sponge and scratch the paintwork.

PUFFING AWAY

If you smoke in your car, the smell will never entirely go.

HOW TO NAIL A TIE DIMPLE

By Mr Mansel Fletcher, Features Editor, MR PORTER

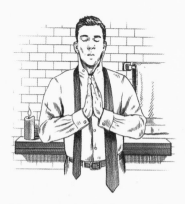

AS A STUDENT I was once invited to a gallery opening, which provided me with a rare opportunity to wear a jacket and tie. As I dressed I took a moment to finesse my tie knot and proudly showed the resulting dimple to my girlfriend. She scoffed and asked who cared about such things, but I was later vindicated when, at the gallery, an older woman complimented me on the fact that my tie bore a pleasing dimple. My affection for tie dimples, unlike my relationship with the girl, has persisted.

Before practical techniques are considered it's important to understand the philosophy of the tie dimple, which is that it should be a personal expression of artful imperfection. It's for men hoping to project an image of *sprezzatura*. *Sprezzatura* implies an element of artifice, so it's crucial to finesse the tie dimple with a natural carelessness, even while the decision to create it is deliberate.

STAND AT EASE

Relax and breathe, because a nonchalant dimple cannot be achieved if you're stressed. We're going to tie a four-in-hand knot, but the creation of a dimple remains the same whatever kind of knot you choose. Here goes. Put the tie around your neck so that the front blade hangs down on your left side, and is a bit longer than the back blade (left-handers may want to reverse this and further left-right instructions). Some people, whose opinions count, like to place the tie and then fold down the collar before they fasten the top button.

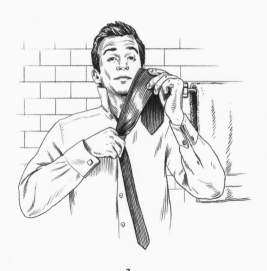

2

TYING THE KNOT

Lay the front blade over the back blade, and then, gripping the tie with your left hand so that your thumb is against the back of the back blade, and your first finger ends up between the two layers of the blades, wrap it once around the back blade. Bring the front blade up behind the knot and flick it over the top.

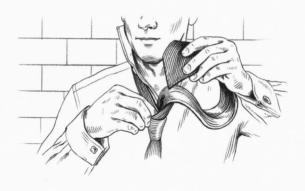

3
THE TIE DIMPLE

Stuff the front blade down the gap that your first finger is keeping open. How tight you pull the knot will affect the shape of the dimple. If you pinch either side of the front blade as you pull it down through the knot you'll end up with a dimple in or near the middle. As you slide the knot up into the collar gap, push the first finger on your left hand into the knot, where it meets the front blade. You should now have a tie dimple.

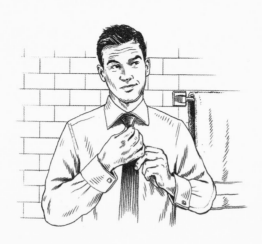

4
GOING TO GREAT LENGTHS

You may want to adjust the dimple, so please do this quickly and while thinking about something else. A good dimple should exude nonchalance and not look too "done". Check you're happy with the lengths of the two blades. It's best if the front blade doesn't extend beyond your waistband. I like the two lengths to be different, which means the rear blade is slightly longer than the front blade. This upsets some people, but none whose distress need concern us.

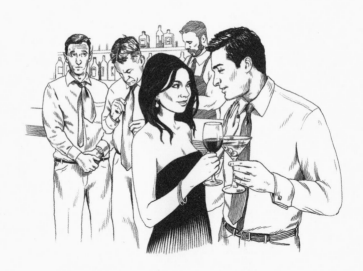

5
KNOW YOUR AUDIENCE

Try pulling the rear blade around towards the front so that it becomes more visible. How far you take this depends, as ever, on what pleases your eye, and where you're going. What's right for a drinks party may not be appropriate for a board meeting.

SOME COMMON MISTAKES

THE WRONG WIDTH

The narrower a tie, the harder it is to create a dimple – it's a real challenge to get a dimple into a tie that's only 6cm wide.

THE WRONG MATERIAL

Very light cotton ties may be too soft to hold a dimple.

THE WRONG KNOT

The chunky and aggressive Windsor knot is incompatible with the nonchalant mood conjured by an elegant dimple.

TRYING TOO HARD

Finessing a tie dimple with all the intensity of an origami master with OCD will not produce what you're looking for.

THE WRONG DESIGN

The world's most elegant knot will be wasted on an ugly tie.

THE WRONG IMPLEMENT

Use your finger to create a dimple. Do not use a dimple maker.

USING THE KEEPER

Many ties have a loop of fabric behind the front blade through which you can tuck the rear blade. Style isn't something that can be pinned down like a dead butterfly; movement is a vital part of it.

HOW TO BE A MAN IN
A BEAR ENCOUNTER

By Mr Frank Miniter, author of The New York Times
bestseller The Ultimate Man's Survival Guide

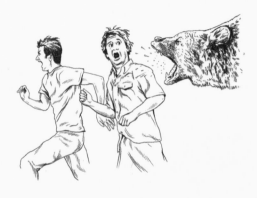

NOW, IF YOU'RE THINKING, "Bear attack, what are the odds?" the answer is: going up all the time. In fact, in North America alone there are more than 750,000 black bears and more than 55,000 grizzlies. It's an environmental success story, of course, but it also means those of us who like to trek have to prepare for encounters.

When you happen upon a bear in the forest, you've stumbled into a test reminiscent of that found in *The Short Happy Life of Francis Macomber* (if you don't know this story by Ernest Hemingway, acquaint yourself; it's manly as hell). Over the years I've been false charged by black bears twice and had quite a few grizzlies growl at me. The key to staying manly in such primal moments is knowing what to do and of course, what not to do. Here are a few pointers.

1
DON'T RUN AWAY SCREAMING

Don't base your knowledge of bears on the old joke: "No, you don't understand", the skinny man says to the fat man. "I don't have to outrun the bear, I just have to outrun you." Turning your back and running from a bear – especially if you scream like a little girl – may trigger a bear's predatory instincts. Hold your ground and back away slowly.

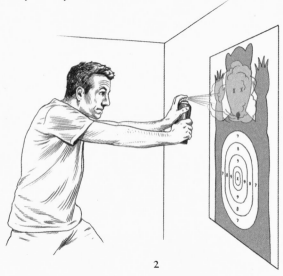

2
PRACTISE MAKES PERFECT

I've worked with Mike Madel, a 30-year veteran grizzly bear specialist. He uses a Karelian bear dog to ward off grizzlies, deters bold bears with rubber bullets and has the unfortunate task of killing problem bears. Yet he also swears by bear spray, and a can is always on his hip. His advice: "Aim low and then bring it up into their face. Keep spraying until the bear turns. And carry a spare." You have to practise. If you think you can read directions on the side of a can as a bear charges, good luck.

3
BEAR SPRAY ISN'T LIKE BUG SPRAY

I was on the Aniak River in Alaska fishing for salmon with brown bears. I ran into a few hikers who smelled so much like pepper I got a spicy chilli craving. I asked what they'd been eating. I soon learnt they'd sprayed bear spray on their packs – they were all flavoured up for the bears. Bear spray (sometimes called pepper spray) uses capsicum and is made to spray into a charging bear's face. It works. But not like bug spray. Get some and make sure you holster it on your belt.

4
HANG YOUR FOOD

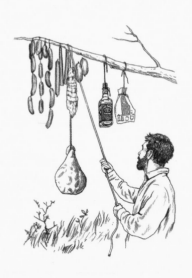

Unless you want to have a bear looking for a way into your tent, hang food or dirty dishes in a tree 50m or more from your camp. Select a pair of branches that are 4 to 5m apart and 4 to 5m high. Attach one end of a rope to a fist-sized rock and tie the other end to a tree trunk. Toss the rock over both branches in succession. Tie a knotted loop in the cord midway between the branches. Attach the food bag (a sealed, waterproof sack) with a slipknot. Pull on the unsecured end of the cord to lift the bag about 3m up. Tie it off.

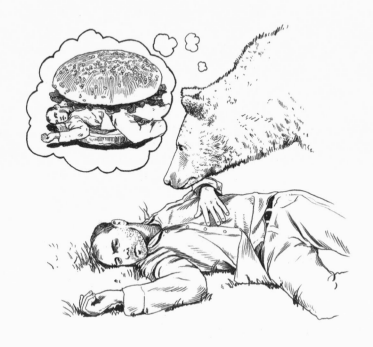

5
KNOW WHEN TO FIGHT

OK, you see a bear. Pull out your bear spray and stay calm. Black bears are mainly docile and just a few attack people each year. But when they do attack they're predatory, so playing dead is just saying, "Eat me". Any bear that attacks at night should be considered predatory. The time to play dead is when you're dealing with a sow protecting her cubs and your bear spray hasn't worked. Black bears are great climbers – you won't get away by climbing a tree – while mature grizzlies are poor climbers. Loud noises can dissuade a bear from attacking. Banging pots together has worked for a lot of people.

SOME COMMON MISTAKES

1

"Look, a bear. Let's go feed it."

2

"Oh, those rangers are always hanging bear warning signs. I can ignore them." A man was killed in Wyoming who did this.

3

"I'll just leave this sandwich right next to my sleeping bag in case I want a midnight snack."

4

"Bear attack? The odds are greater that I'll be hit by lightning." Actually, when you go where bears are, your odds increase. By comparison, if you like whitewater kayaking, then your odds of drowning are not the national average.

5

"I'll just leave my can of bear spray in the car for safekeeping." The cans are aerosols. Their contents will expand in a hot car and might even explode.

HOW TO BUY A ROLEX

*By Mr James Dowling, Rolex historian and co-author
of* The Best of Time: Rolex Wristwatches

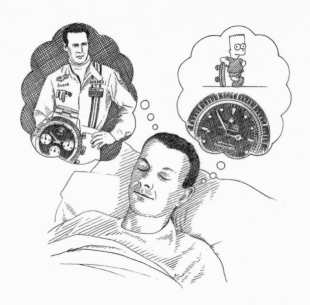

SO YOU WANT TO buy a Rolex. The reasons are irrelevant – perhaps you were in Milan and liked the way the suave locals were wearing them, or maybe you just got a nice bonus. Regardless, once you have made the decision, you are likely to start some online research. The next thing you know, you feel seriously overwhelmed and out of your depth. Relax! Just stick to these sure-fire tips and then you can enjoy your expertly considered Rolex.

KNOW YOUR STYLE

Ultimately, no one can tell you exactly which Rolex model is best for you. The right piece for you is one that you like and that suits your lifestyle. If you wear a suit most days, there's one model that is a classic choice; if you dress more casually, there's another model for you. Rolex has been around for more than a century and has produced hundreds of models, but I will simplify it for you: if you are part of the first group (suit wearer), buy a Datejust; if the second (casual dresser), buy a Submariner.

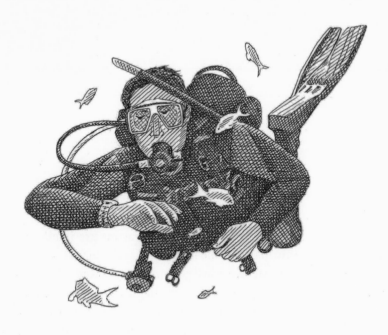

2
LEARN THE LEXICON

On the faces of both of these watches, look below "Rolex" for these crucial words: "Oyster" or "Perpetual". "Oyster" means that it is waterproof – Datejusts can go down to 50m and Submariners four times that. "Perpetual" means that the watch winds itself as you wear it, so it's important to ask how recently the watch has been serviced. A mechanical watch needs to be serviced every three years. If it hasn't been serviced it may not wind itself correctly.

3
FIGURE IT OUT

So how much should you pay for a vintage Rolex? Datejusts can be found from approximately £1,750/ €2,000/ $2,800, Submariners from around £2,500/ €3,000/ $4,000. Expect to pay more if the watch has sapphire rather than plastic covering the dial. Sapphire is much harder to scratch, but plastic has more of a vintage look.

4
BUY FOR LOVE

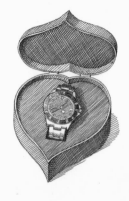

Don't confuse a brand-new Rolex with an investment. The truth is most Rolex watches drop in value the moment you leave the shop, which is why buying vintage can be a good deal. A vintage Rolex will almost certainly recoup the price you paid if you keep it for three to five years.

BUY FOR NOW

Who knows if the brand-new Rolex you buy will become the sought-after, valuable model of the future? No one, so never believe anyone who says they do. Only time will tell if your watch will turn out to be the greatest investment you've ever made. As long as it's the greatest watch you ever buy, it's a win-win situation either way.

SOME COMMON MISTAKES

FALLING TOO QUICKLY

You may fall for, or obsess over, the first Rolex you see, and want to buy it immediately. Don't. Rolex made more than half a million watches in each of the past 25 years alone. Do your research, bide your time and find a source you trust – it will be worth the wait.

ACTING ON LOOKS ALONE

Don't enter into a marriage that will never work. Sometimes you will find a 1980s watch with a 1970s dial, or a Submariner with a bracelet that was only ever used on other models. While it may be attractive, it will be hard to resell and once you know the truth, it will irritate you every time you glance at your wrist.

NOT PUTTING THE HOURS IN

There are dozens and dozens of books on Rolex watches and even more websites. Take your time, read up and talk to dealers and other collectors before taking the plunge. No hour spent on research is a wasted hour.

HOW TO TAKE THE
PERFECT PENALTY

By Dr Ken Bray, author of How to Score:
Science and the Beautiful Game

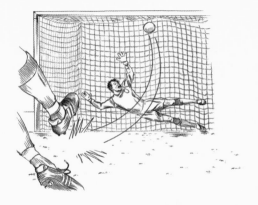

WE ASKED Dr Ken Bray, a renowned sport scientist and
theoretical physicist for some tips on taking a football penalty...
So: you've just been awarded a penalty kick and you're going to take
it. Or your team has fought its way through to a shoot-out and your
name's on the list of penalty takers. Anxious? You should be. You're
about to face one of the most testing physical and psychological
encounters in sport. And no matter whether you play for your pub
team or the national side, there will be nerves. But as someone
once said, it's not a question of having butterflies, but getting them
all flying in formation. Follow these key steps to ensure success.

I
KEEP YOUR FOCUS AT JUST THE RIGHT LEVEL

Jog, don't walk, to the penalty spot. You want to keep the right level of adrenaline flowing and brisk movement helps calm the nerves and maintain what sports scientists call "psychological arousal". Just outside the penalty area, slow to a walk and breathe deeply. Pick up the ball, spin it a few times, then stamp down on any damage, imaginary or real, around the penalty spot. Place the ball with care, then make eye contact with the goalie for a second or so. You must stay in control of the psychological encounter: your mantra is "my ball, my penalty".

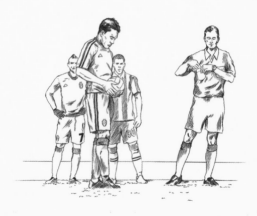

2
DEALING WITH DIFFICULT GOALKEEPERS

Of course the goalie needn't go along with this and might play you at your own game. Let's say he leaves the goal line and approaches you to engage in some friendly banter. His objective is to destroy your focus and to emphasise just how tall and agile he is. Don't be drawn: place your foot on the ball and wait until the ref orders him back to the goal line. Then go through your "spin the ball, repair the damage routine". Make him wait. Your ball, your penalty.

3
FOCUS, FOCUS, FOCUS

You now walk back to your run-up position and wait for the ref's whistle. The goalie will be madly cavorting about, but it's quite legal as long as he stays on the goal line. It's just another attempt to destroy your concentration. Look at the target area of the goal where you intend to place your shot. Try to visualise the shot you will execute in your mind's eye. Sports psychologists call this technique "imaging". It's a powerful way of concentrating your focus, and blotting out the surrounding stressful elements.

4
HITTING THE SPOT

Even the best goalies have a finite reach (*see below*). Aiming inside the envelope is risky because about 50% of penalties hit here are saved. Conversely, 80% of penalties aimed into the "unsaveable zone" succeed. Your optimum shot should be shoulder height, played to the goalie's left or right. Avoid those parts of the unsaveable zone close to the ground and near the goalposts as the margin for error is greater. Remember: you don't have to knock the skin off the ball. "Place with pace" is what you should be thinking.

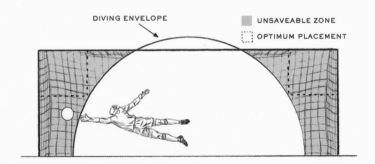

DIVING ENVELOPE | UNSAVEABLE ZONE
OPTIMUM PLACEMENT

SOME COMMON MISTAKES

FAILING TO PREPARE

It's many years since an England coach argued that practising penalties was unnecessary. Hone your technique by taking spot kicks after hard training sessions. Don't shoot at an empty net. It's important to have a goalie in place to achieve maximum realism.

TAKE A PROPER RUN-UP

Don't take a single step back and imagine that you'll beat a wily goalkeeper with a nonchalant swing of your boot at the ball. Control of direction and pace of shot are vital and it's much easier to achieve the ideal combination from a short, purposeful run-up.

NEVER CHANGE YOUR MIND

Deliver the shot you've practised, the one you should be "imaging" before the ref blows his whistle for the kick. Why gamble with an unrehearsed shot? Worst of all is a decision to change tactics during the run-up itself: easily the most common cause of missed penalties in the coaching manual.

HOW TO DE-BILBO YOUR FEET THIS SUMMER

By Ms Jodie Harrison, Editor, MR PORTER

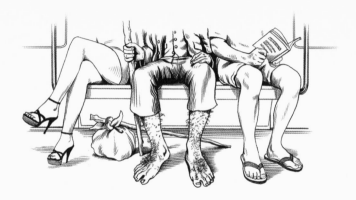

SUMMERTIME. A time for festivals, alfresco dining and flagrant foot flaunting. But after months of forcing them to exist in conditions similar to, say, mushrooms or insect larvae, are your feet now up to public airing? Probably not. Summer commuting on the subway or bus offers people an inordinate amount of free time to stare directly at your feet. Women *can* and *will* scrutinise every bump, crustacean and outcrop. So, why not prevent any awkward glances with a little pre-emptive preening? Here, we've compiled some viable tips to get your feet looking more human than hobbit and help you to shape them into the perfect backdrop for that new pair of beach-friendly sandals.

1
BE HONEST

Start off by looking at your feet with the same critical eye you would offer up to say, an undercooked burger from a street vendor or a suspiciously stained chair in your student nephew's flat. Would you allow your child to touch them without risking a life-changing ailment? No? Then for goodness sake keep them away from the public. If there is still a chance of saving them, read on.

2
SCRUB UP

As when cleaning a fine pair of John Lobb shoes, the first thing to do here is soften the skin in preparation. Take a long shower or bath, allowing enough soaking time to soften any rough skin on your heels and balls of your feet. Then, using a body scrub or foot scrub, massage them for five minutes and rinse. Finish by trimming your nails (straight across and not too short). Then give your nails and cuticles a good but gentle scrub with a nail brush.

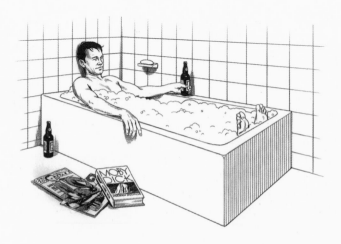

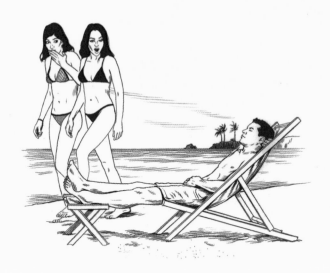

3
DE-FLUFF, DE-FUZZ AND DESCALE

When it comes to dead skin on your feet, the best removal device comes in the form of a professional foot file. If they are unappealing, hairy and Bilbo-like, it might be worth considering a few rounds of laser hair removal, a treatment that works by directing intense pulsed light on the area of the hair itself, destroying the follicle.

4
NAIL THE ISSUE

Yellowing, cankerous toenails make you look like an old man. Black bruised nails, the result of trauma (a pooling of blood beneath the nail usually common in football- or marathon-inclined men), are equally off-putting. If your nail colour doesn't improve get it checked out with a podiatrist (not a pedicurist – that's the type your wife visits for a repaint).

POWDER YOUR TOES

Reducing friction between your foot, sock and shoe will result in generally more attractive feet – as recommended by foot specialist Mr Bastien Gonzalez: "I use talcum powder to absorb the humidity at night and only the following day will I put a shoetree in the shoe, once it's really dried out. I also use another sprinkle each time I go to use them. It reduces any friction." When it comes to your talcum powder, choose one which is exceptionally fine in quality and preferably with an attractive fragrance.

SOME COMMON MISTAKES

BELIEVING IT NOT TO MATTER

I once met a woman who left a man due to the appearance of his feet and the fact that they used to touch hers in bed. Sure she was a callous, shallow woman, but this tale still serves as a warning. Ignore your feet and she might just love you a little bit less.

WEARING SOCKS WITH YOUR SANDALS

Certain designers may still unleash this chin-scratching styling trick at fashion shows but this is real life, and no man should ever be seen in this ensemble.

WEARING SHOES REPEATEDLY

Men with large shoe collections will rarely have bad feet, because if you wear the same pair over and over again without letting the perspiration dry out, your feet and shoes are basically rotting.

HOW TO CHOP LIKE A PRO

*By Mr Yoshinori Ishii, executive chef
of Michelin-starred Umu, London*

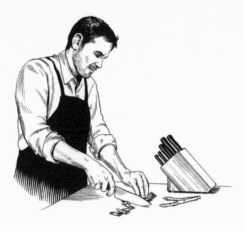

FOR ANYONE wanting to be a pro at this, you must practise. If you do it for long enough, you'll be able to chop with your eyes closed, scale thickness with the fingers of your left hand, and feel texture with your right. The key points to remember are pretty universal: use a good knife, slide smoothly, and use the whole section of the knife.

When I learnt my knife skills in Japan, I started with *katsura-muki*, one of the most difficult yet key cutting techniques for professional Japanese chefs. It is used for making very thin ribbons of vegetables. When I started learning culinary skills, I made sure to practise every night after I finished dinner service. Although I've been a chef for 20 years, I practise every day in order to maintain the sensitivity of my fingers and the condition of my knives.

I

TOOL UP

Choose the correct knife depending on your dexterity and which foods you are planning to cut. Before buying knives, look at how much steel is in the knife. Look for any signs of joining or welding, particularly in the hilt. This is a weak point. The best knives are made from a single piece of Swedish steel. The material of the edge has to be very high quality – which you can get with most well-known knife makers. For the Japanese specialist, the best knives are made from a single piece of iron and are called *honyaki*.

2

PREPARE YOUR WEAPON

Every time you use a knife, be sure to use a sharpening stone first – which you can get easily from a kitchen equipment shop. I got my sharpening stone made by a Japanese ceramics company. Make sure you soak the stone in water for a while before use. Not only will this give you the best edge; it'll also remove the least amount of material.

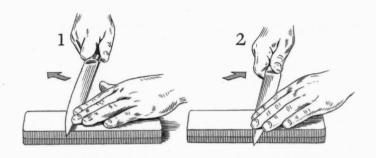

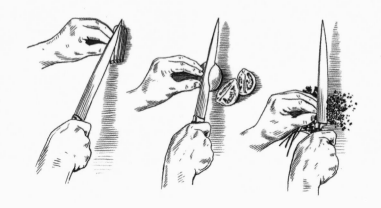

3
HOW TO CUT IT

When cutting something, you have to slide the blade for as long as possible. The key is not to press. The blade of a chef's knife is divided into three sections: the tip, the midsection and the base. Use the tip, or pointed end of the knife, to cut evenly spaced slices. Use the midsection of the knife for general slicing, such as vegetables and for cutting apples into wedges. Use the section closest to the knife handle when chopping herbs or fine ingredients. When slicing meat, use the mid to top sections. When chopping meat, the section closest to the knife handle is best.

4
PRACTISE MAKES PERFECT

To become a pro, you have to practise cutting the same ingredients every day so the knife will become comfortable in your hand. Try to do this as often as possible, just as a soccer player practises each day with his ball.

5
KEEP YOUR DIGITS

Remember to keep the fingers of your guiding hand curled under to prevent cutting yourself. When I started to use knives, I cut my finger quite often. Currently, after more than 20 years of practise, it still happens – but only rarely!

SOME COMMON MISTAKES

CHEAP EQUIPMENT

Since kitchen knives will be an investment that are used daily, selecting good durable ones that handle well is crucial.

A POOR SELECTION

Choosing the incorrect knife for a specific food just won't cut it.

BLUNT INSTRUMENTS

Cutting with a dull knife is more dangerous than using a very sharp one – the knife can slip off the food rather than cut into it easily.

SHARING YOUR TOOLS

Sharing knives with your housemates or family is a mistake. Different knife shapes suit different people.

BEING LAZY

Practise makes perfect. The more you chop, the better you'll become.

THE KNACK

HOW TO ACE A BEST MAN'S SPEECH

By Mr Dan Davies, editor of Esquire Weekly, *and newly wed*

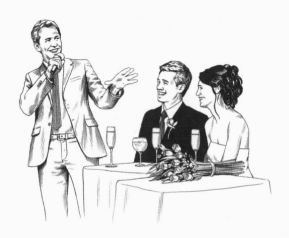

FOR ANY MAN facing up to the challenge of representing his closest friend on the biggest day of his life, watching the opening scene of the British comedy *I Give it a Year* should be at the top of any pre-wedding check list. In it, the hapless buffoon played by Mr Stephen Merchant delivers possibly the most toe-curling best man's speech. It's so bad that not even the groom can disguise his horror. Whatever people say about this being the most supportive audience you'll ever face, the best man's speech is a tightrope. You will either traverse it successfully and be hailed as the hero who lights the fuse for the fun part of the evening, or you'll fall horribly and want to spend the rest of the wedding hiding in the loo. So do yourself a favour, and take heed of the following advice...

I
PREPARE FOR SUCCESS

You might fancy yourself as a raconteur, but being poorly prepared is the pathway to disaster. Do the groundwork: canvass the groom's circle of friends, his family and his wife-to-be for funny, insightful anecdotes. Make a few notes, but don't feel obliged to write out the speech longhand, because reading it out may sound stilted.

2
BE HONEST ABOUT YOUR ABILITY
TO RAISE A LAUGH

"It's been an emotional day. Even the cake is in tiers." Would this make you laugh? No. Every best man's speech gag recommended on the internet is either dismal or inappropriate. Avoid at all costs – it's much better to stick to amusing true stories.

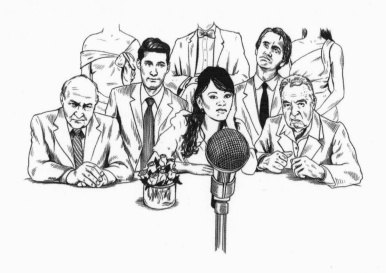

3
CHECK THE GUESTS CAN HEAR YOU

How often do you use a microphone? Hmm, thought so. Ensure everyone can hear you by testing the volume with your impersonation of the man who introduces heavyweight boxing. Or just ask if everyone can hear you. Either way, look up while you're speaking to engage the audience and project your voice.

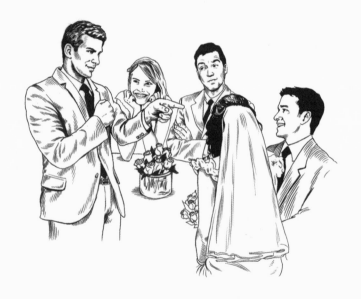

4
BE HEARTFELT

Give examples of what a great guy the groom is, tell him how wonderful his new bride is, and how happy you are for him. Do not refer to former conquests, ex-girlfriends, embarrassing ailments, brushes with the law and any form of substance abuse. It's your job to make him sound, and feel, good – not to humiliate him.

5
ENJOY A WELL-DESERVED DRINK, OR TWO

Kick back, relax and enjoy the free-flowing alcohol, but not until after you've given the speech. Delivering a best man's speech is stressful and a wedding day is a long one, so it's vital to pace yourself. If you're not feeling nervous you've overdone it at the bar. If this is the case, falling over on your way back to your chair is likely to raise the only laugh you'll get all night.

SOME COMMON MISTAKES

HUMILIATING THE GROOM

As best man your job is to support your friend throughout an exciting but stressful day. Neither he, nor anybody else, wants to hear about the appalling, tawdry things that went down on that "legendary" university rugby tour.

SPEAKING IN RIDDLES

If it's bad to recount unflattering anecdotes it's almost worse to allude to juvenile misadventures without revealing what they are. Try to entertain the whole wedding party, not just the guys who were at the stag night.

TALKING FOR TOO LONG

Keep it short and sweet – five minutes is perfect. People want to hear what you have to say, but go on too long and their thoughts will turn to dinner, or their wish for another drink. It's best to leave them wanting more.

THE KNACK

HOW TO TWEET

*By Mr Peter Serafinowicz, member of the tweet elite
and author of* A Billion Jokes (Volume One)

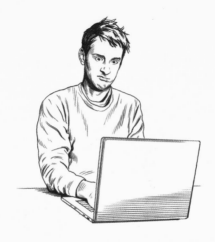

SET UP in March 2006 by California-based Mr Jack Dorsey, Twitter has more than 500 million users, with around 340 million tweets sent a day. The quickest way to spread knowledge and news to the world, it has changed the way we think, work and communicate. Quick-fire and free, however, it can also be excruciatingly banal. From meaningless missives about the weather to 140-character lunch descriptions, it's easy to be an insufferable tweeter. Or, if you're careless, a libellous one. London-based comedian, writer and director Mr Peter Serafinowicz has gained more than 650,000 followers by being a master of wit and intrigue. Here, he reveals how he's become a member of the tweet elite.

1

CHOOSE YOUR USP

When I first started using Twitter, I had no idea what to do. I linked to a couple of things, said hello. Pretty soon I'd settled into a joke thing – using Twitter as a conduit for all the stupid ideas that appear in my brain, which normally would have no outlet. But everyone's different. Of course you'll be influenced by other people, as with any form of expression, but try to be you. If it comes from the heart, it goes to the heart.

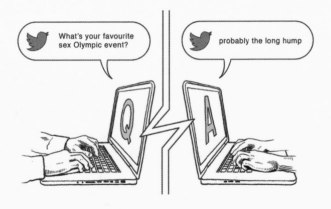

2

DON'T BE AFRAID

Tweet different content and try various things. I do Q&A sessions on Twitter known as #PSQA. Someone suggests a topic and I try to come up with witty answers. I get thousands of replies and scan through them for any that I can think of a funny answer to. It's daunting, and often my first answer is not that great, but it jump-starts me, and then it becomes easier. Dive in! NB: using features such as Twitpic can be fun, but never post a picture of your genitals.

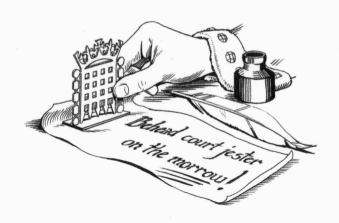

3
GET YOUR NEWS FROM TWITTER

The latest stories always break on Twitter well before any news websites. Also, you get to see lots of scandalous stuff that doesn't make it anywhere else. Twitter uses hashtags #likethis to make things easier to search, and allow popular topics to trend. This tradition dates back to medieval times when kings would place a tiny portcullis next to things they wanted to remember.

4
PLAY NICE

Twitter is usually a pretty polite, self-regulating place, however, if someone is mean to you it's simple to block them, and then for you they cease to exist. Don't be horrible to people! If you're replying to someone using their @name, they can see it in their timeline, and you are directly communicating with them. Again, don't be @ d**k. Choose your name carefully. Mine is @serafinowicz, which annoys my brother.

5
KEEP IT SHORT

Hack away at your sentence to strip away all the flesh from the skeleton. Especially if you're writing a joke. Concise, clear and short sentences make more of an impact. Shakespeare said "Brevity is the soul of wit." He later amended it to Brevit, before finally settling on B=LOL.

SOME COMMON MISTAKES

NARROW-MINDEDNESS

Follow lots of people, and not just "celebrities". There are so many interesting, funny people out there – if you like someone, check out who they follow, and follow them.

FORGETTING TO SELF-SENSOR

Some people can be sensitive to strong language and may unfollow you if you use profanities. So don't f**k up.

LACK OF CLARITY

A good and sturdy general rule (or maxim) when writing is to keep sentences as concise, clear and non-verbose as you possibly can, avoiding digressions, distractions, tautologies and tautologies.

TWITTER ADDICTION

Try to experience the real world, too. It's pretty nice! The graphics, in particular, are amazing.

HOW TO BUY LINGERIE FOR A LADY

By Ms Jodie Harrison, Editor, MR PORTER

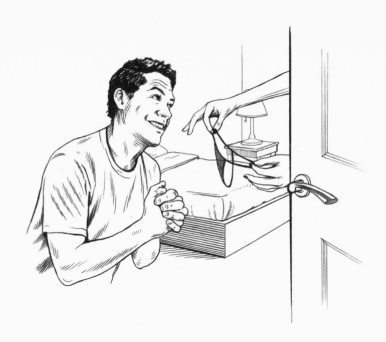

IT'S YOUR FIRST anniversary together. You're enjoying the haze of new-found affection and lust, and as such, lingerie seems like the perfectly pitched gesture. You aim for something chic and expensive. You leave with overpriced dental floss that spends the rest of its short life stuffed into a drawer. You got it wrong. Again. Next time, here's how you get it right.

I

SEXY = UNWEARABLE

This is the big hole most men fall down when buying lingerie. As crazy as it sounds, sexy panties or bras can also be comfortable enough to wear day to day, you just have to choose carefully. If you want her to actually wear what you've bought, go for a black or white, reasonably stretchy fabric that's not going to sever her spleen every time she attempts to put a pair of jeans on. Designers such as Kiki De Montparnasse are our go-to choice for lingerie.

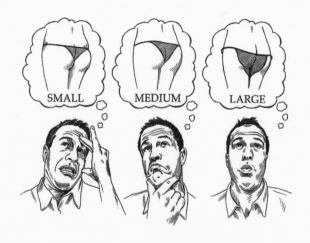

SMALL   MEDIUM   LARGE

2

PANTS RESEARCH

When it comes to knickers, go for a medium unless you absolutely, categorically know differently. Unlike the reverse scenario, buying large isn't exactly a complimentary gesture. Similarly, buying a size that's way too small just seems either a little lazy or too keen to please. Make like Goldilocks and go for something *juuuuust* right. If that fails, try something less size-specific, such as a silk robe or nightdress.

3
STYLE NOTES

As a clean, straight-leg-A.P.C.-jeans kind of man, you probably wouldn't welcome distressed bootlegs making an appearance on your birthday. It's a style thing, so take notes on her current lingerie preferences. This isn't the time to mould your beloved into a ball-stamping, *Fifty Shades*-style sex mistress when she's more of a "tea, biscuits and a good book" gal. Unless she's expressed a desire to slut it up in the bedroom, don't go for all leather and lace.

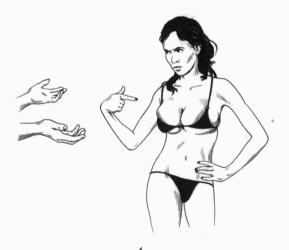

4
BRAND TO BRAND

Like railway companies, lingerie designers seem to find a perverse sort of pleasure in providing products and services vastly different to one another. One brand's Ms Kate Moss' cups can be another's Ms Dolly Parton's. Researching the labels she actually opts for in her own lingerie collection will alleviate any sizing miscalculations and ensuing embarrassment. So get rooting in her drawers, as it were, and make notes.

CHECK YOUR AUDIENCE

Nipple tassels, waspies, whips, peekaboo bras or any sort of restraining devices should not be unwrapped in front of an audience. You may think such a gift makes you look as if you have an enviable sex life but, actually, it just makes you seem a little gross. Lingerie is a personal gift, meant for personal gifting scenarios. Choose your moment wisely.

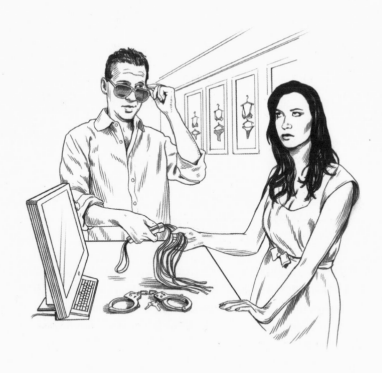

SOME COMMON MISTAKES

SALES GIRL BLINKERS

Underwear shopping can be embarrassing and for some cruel reason, the person you come face to face with is usually unfeasibly hot. Don't let your trousers or her charms lead you in the wrong direction. Research and buy online so you won't get distracted.

SPECIAL FORCES

If she's ample up top, then she'll need an underwired bra. If she has more than enough, the service of specific brands will be required (Elle Macpherson Intimates and Stella McCartney go all the way up to E, F and G cups). Whatever you do, avoid anything that calls itself a "soft cup". These little beauties are more suited to barely-there types.

GETTING TECHNICAL

If you can't figure out what strap, clasp or clip goes where, chances are she won't either. If it's got more strings and things than a cat's cradle, I can pretty much guarantee it will be worn once and then never see the light of day again. Simple is often sexiest.

SIZE MATTERS

Men tend to think small when it comes to buying lingerie. Whether this is wishful thinking, a misjudged sort of kindness or an innate inability to gauge size and distance (wink, wink) remains a mystery to women the world over. Whatever the cause, stop it. Use your head. SpongeBob SquarePants wouldn't fit into Patrick Star's shorts and attempting to make him fit would be humiliating. Point made.

HOW TO MIX A DRINK FOR HER

By Mr Barrie Wilson, cocktail expert for Diageo

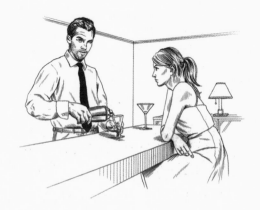

THERE ARE FOUR things the modern gentleman should be able to do: change a tyre, tie a bow tie, start a fire and, most importantly, mix a great cocktail. You may feel that the latter is probably the most difficult to achieve, but with a little practise and a lot more confidence – this could prove to be a valuable and impressive tool.

There are many classic cocktails you could choose from to be part of your repertoire (see page 160 for my personal favourite), but for maximum effect you need to make a bespoke creation that reflects whoever you're trying to impress. Learn your guest's favourite fruits, herbs, juices and spirits and get to work on a cocktail that you can name after her. This will show that you are a great listener, and ensures your bar at home is the only venue that will serve her favourite cocktail.

I
TRUST YOUR TOOLS

Select the cocktail equipment that you are comfortable using; there is nothing worse than a shaker exploding all over you and your guest. Also, if you use a two-piece shaker, these can sometimes be tricky to separate. Get practising and make it all look incredibly slick.

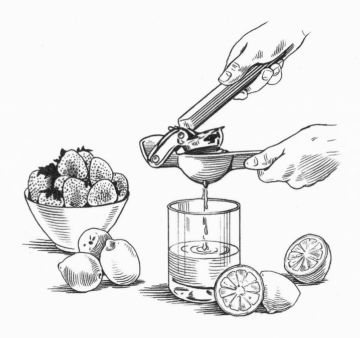

2
THE FINER DETAILS

Make sure you have fresh, seasonal fruit. Pre-squeezed fresh lemon or lime juice will save time and mess. Also, make sure you have something for a sweet tooth; sugar syrup, agave nectar, honey or elderflower cordial should always be in your cupboard.

3
ICE UP

Don't assume you can make cocktails with the ice tray in your freezer – this is not enough. You will need a big bag of ice. No one wants a warm drink, and it's better to have too much than run out.

4
EYE CONTACT

When you are shaking your cocktail, make sure you never make eye contact with your guest. You usually have to shake for 10 seconds – which can get extremely uncomfortable even if you share a glance.

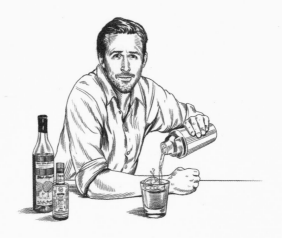

5
DON'T DO A GOSLING

In *Crazy Stupid Love*, Mr Ryan Gosling mixes an old fashioned. This is one of the more alcoholic cocktails. The aim isn't to get her drunk – she needs to remember your skills, so make sure you keep the cocktail light, avoiding overly alcoholic concoctions.

SOME COMMON MISTAKES

BAD BALANCE

Make sure you get the correct balance of sweet versus sour. If you get this right, the cocktail should taste like a sorbet. If anything, make it more on the sweet side, as it is generally more palatable than a sour drink.

OVER EGGING

Using egg white in a drink is only for aesthetics and texture. If you can taste it then you have used too much – it will be chalky and unpleasant. Only use approximately 5-10ml per drink.

FRUIT FAIL

Never ever buy citrus juice pre-made in a bottle; nothing is more delicious than freshly squeezed. Also, you can play around with your sour of choice – why not use pink grapefruit instead of lemon or lime?

ALCOHOLIC TENDENCIES

Strong drinks are lovely if they are made correctly, but generally you can only have the one glass. A good rule of thumb should be that no drink exceeds two units of alcohol, which equates to 50ml of alcohol per drink.

FLAMBOYANT DECORATION

Don't make the garnish too elaborate. The star of the show should always be the drink; the garnish should be simple, rustic and serve a purpose. No cocktail umbrellas and sparklers, please.

A FAIL-SAFE COCKTAIL FOR HER

THE MERCER SOUR

This is perfect as it is light, flavoursome and smooth. Served on the rocks in a tumbler, it is a delicious drink you can both enjoy.

INGREDIENTS	EQUIPMENT
1/8th honeydew melon	Knife
1 kiwi fruit	Chopping board
50ml Tanqueray gin	Two-piece Parisian shaker
25ml fresh lemon juice	Muddler
20ml sugar syrup	Lemon squeezer
5ml egg white	Old-fashioned tumbler
Ice	Hawthorne strainer

STEP 1

Chop the melon into wedges and place in the shaker. Cut a wheel from the kiwi and set aside. With the remaining fruit, drop only the flesh into the shaker. Using the muddler, squash the fruit until soft.

STEP 2

Add the Tanqueray and squeeze the juice of half a lemon into the shaker, then add the sugar syrup and the egg white. In order to emulsify the egg white you should shake this first without ice; do this for 10 seconds, then add the ice and shake hard.

STEP 3

Fill your glass with ice and use the strainer to pour the liquid over the ice; you should have a lovely creamy head to the drink. Finally add the wheel of kiwi fruit to the top of the drink to garnish.

MR DAVID BOWIE

We pay tribute to the original
pop chameleon

Words by Mr Dylan Jones, editor-in-chief of British *GQ*

MR DAVID BOWIE swirls around us like dry ice, always has done, pretty much always will. I was walking by *GQ*'s art department and I saw a copy of *Isolar II* on someone's desk (if you don't know what *Isolar II* is then I suggest you probably won't want to read the rest of this piece*), and this morning I heard "Where Are We Now?", Mr Bowie's extraordinary comeback single wafting out of a shop doorway as I made my way to work. Magazines and newspapers were full of editorial for the V&A exhibition in early 2013, and everyone and their mother was discussing the album, *The Next Day*, and every old Mr Bowie record from "Space Oddity" to "Everyone Says Hi" is still playing somewhere as I write. Personally I wouldn't have it any other way. I love Mr Bowie, always have done – well, since I was 12 – and not a day goes by when I don't think about him, and of course the way he looks. When Mr Bowie appeared on *Top of the Pops* on Thursday 6 July 1972 with The Spiders from Mars singing "Starman", he had me at "Didn't". Like millions of other teenagers in the UK that evening – at that time the show was regularly watched by a quarter of the population – I found his performance genuinely transformative, even though I only saw it in black and white. Unlike those who claimed they saw the Sex Pistols at The Screen on the Green in Islington, London, everyone who claimed they saw Mr Bowie on *Top of the Pops* was probably telling the truth. I saw the broadcast sitting alone in the sitting room of our three-up, three-down semi in Deal, Kent, on an otherwise unremarkable summer's evening.

And, having seen him, I went out and tried to emulate his haircut. It appeared to me that his hair was the element that personified Mr Bowie, and in this respect I was uncharacteristically ahead of the curve. You weren't going to get hordes of teenage boys and girls wandering around my town centre dressed in the kind of get-up that he wore on television, although it was completely logical that they – we, us – could all copy his haircut. Except that it wasn't "me" at all, and it was always "they". I wasn't cool, wasn't in with the in-crowd and the terms on which they acknowledged and accepted each other in the playground were not terms that had any bearing on me. So if I could get the haircut, then things might begin to change. A successful Bowie haircut could bestow countless wonders on me, or so I thought. My Saturday morning trip to the unisex hairdressers was planned days in advance. I'd scouted the town for the various barbers and hairdressers who might offer this newfangled cut. I went through the local paper looking for more, and methodically called them all up, asking if they indeed did offer a "Bowie cut". Most didn't know what I was talking about, but one said they could probably do what I wanted, so why didn't I come in and they would give me a free consultation. I can't remember exactly what I was wearing when I turned up, but I've got a fair idea it involved a pair of slightly flared plaid trousers or a cheap pair of Oxford bags, a round-collared shirt with a repeated print of a French café scene, and probably an extremely unfashionable canvas jacket, with aircraft carrier lapels and large silver buttons. Years later the French designer Mr Jean Paul Gaultier would say that it's always the badly dressed people who are the most interesting, but in my case he would have been colossally wrong, as I was the prisoner of what I was wearing rather than the proprietor. Consequently it was the

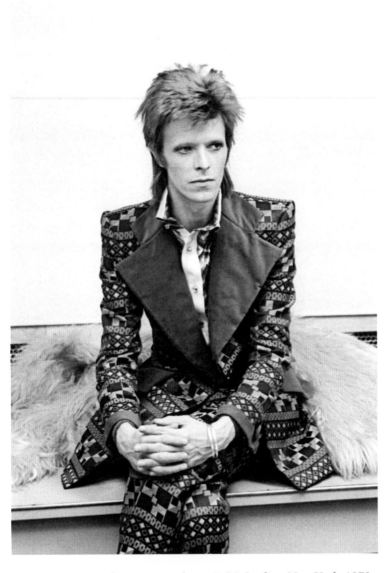

Mr Bowie posing for a portrait shot at RCA Studios, New York, 1973

haircut which was going to save me. It was the haircut that was going to make me not just acceptable, but appealing.

Unsurprisingly, this was not to be. Having walked to the hairdressers at the appointed hour, I sat in the chair and blithely told the stylist what I wanted. And what I wanted was to have hair like Mr Bowie, to have a large quiff on top, with a feather cut beneath, and locks brushing passed the edge of my collar. Tough. "It won't work, 'cause your hair's all wrong," the hairdresser took great delight in telling me. "For this kind of haircut you need hair that goes up, and yours just goes down. No offence, but it just won't work." Which is how I ended up leaving the salon that day with a haircut that approximated the one sported by Mr Dave Hill, the decidedly odd-looking, buck-toothed guitarist in Slade, the one who looked like Cleopatra in nine-eyelet Dr. Martens boots. The clothes would eventually come – fur-collared Budgie jackets, pinstriped high-waisted bags, platform shoes and high-collared shirts – but it was the haircut I wanted more than anything else, the haircut that could have helped me bridge the credibility gap. As it is, I had to wait months for my hair to grow out, and from then until 1977 I kept it shoulder length, parted in the middle. It wasn't until punk came along that I finally got my Bowie cut, in colour if not in shape.

Isolar II was the very trendy post/magazine available on the *Stage* tour

THE REPORT
GROOMING MATTERS

*Read on to identify your type, and
the skin regime that will suit your lifestyle*

Words by Mr Ahmed Zambarakji

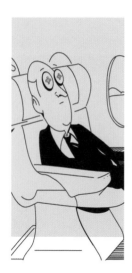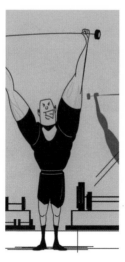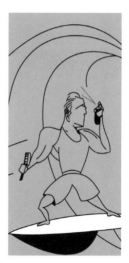

ALL MEN may have been created equal, but that doesn't mean we're all the same. Since the modern man can come in a variety of guises, we've compiled a selection of go-to products suited to a variety of lifestyles. So whether you're an office professional or the kind of man who lives life on the edge, there's no reason your skin shouldn't be as considered as your wardrobe.

While a nine-to-five job is hardly up there in the danger stakes, the office is a quietly aggressive environment. A work week that exceeds 40 hours, exposed to air conditioning and stress, will undermine your appearance. Equip your desk drawer with an instant energiser.

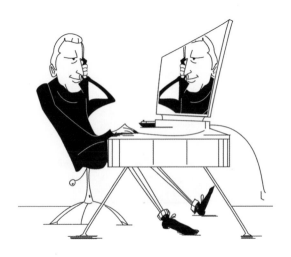

PROBLEM

Tired eyes

SOLUTION

Clinique's foolproof Anti-Fatigue Eye Cooling Gel helps deflate puffy eyes that have grown weary from staring at a computer monitor all day.

THE GYM JUNKIE

No bona fide gym-goer sweats through endless sets of Russian twists without intending to put his hard work on display. Fortunately, there is a grooming product that can help boost the benefits of a rigorous work-out routine.

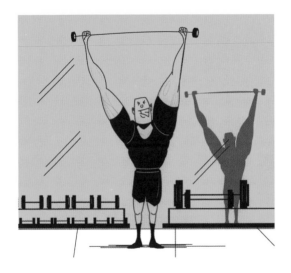

PROBLEM

Stubborn fat that hides shy abs

SOLUTION

NuBo's The 6-Pack Treatment claims to supercharge any abdominal routine by speeding up your metabolism and triggering lipolysis (the body's innate ability to release fat from cells), thus helping to create an intimidatingly ripped midsection.

THE DUDE

A dependable skincare regime probably isn't the first thing that springs to mind given the Dude spends his spare time rolling in dirt and hanging off cliffs. There is, however, a super-strength product that can limit the damage caused by his extreme outdoor pursuits.

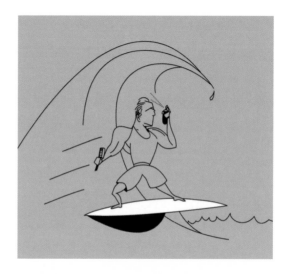

PROBLEM

UV exposure

SOLUTION

Few broad-spectrum sunscreens come more impenetrable than Kiehl's Cross-Terrain UV Face Protector SPF 50, as test-driven by *National Geographic*'s team of young explorers. The waxy formula also happens to be pretty sweat-resistant.

THE SUN LOVER

The glamour of the Sun Lover's year-round tan is undercut by the fact that excessive UV exposure will soon turn his skin into a well-worn sofa. Repairing the damage caused by baking on a lounger is no small feat and requires a serious restorative suncare product.

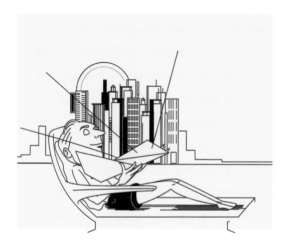

PROBLEM

Sun-induced wrinkles after too much time on the Lilo

SOLUTION

Institut Esthederm's Refreshing After-Sun Fondant can help repair damaged skin tissue and relieve burning – and, crucially, it boosts the Sun Lover's signature perma-tan at the same time.

THE ECO EPICUREAN

Being right-on isn't easy when businesses throw around words such as "ethical" and "organic" without any real proof. The discerning Eco Epicurean will covet brands that have more seals of approvals from stringent regulating boards than you can shake a stick at.

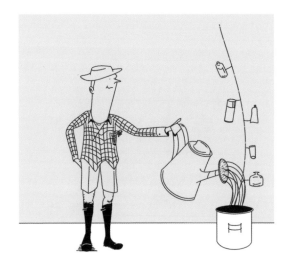

PROBLEM

Sleepy chakras

SOLUTION

There's no doubting the eco-credentials of Intelligent Nutrients' innovative products, especially the food-grade Aromatics, best used as body oils and formulated to wake up your energy levels. The oils can induce specific moods, from "alert" to, ahem, "amorous".

THE JET-SETTER

Even though he may enjoy the luxury of a private aircraft, the Jet-Setter is not exempt from the ravages of air travel. Bouncing back from jet lag while nourishing skin that has been stripped dry at 30,000ft can be achieved with some tactful post-flight grooming.

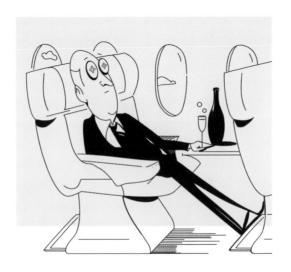

PROBLEM

Red eyes that come with taking the, er, red-eye

SOLUTION

Cabin air does a fine job of sucking the moisture – and charm – out of the Jet-Setter's face. Applied the night you land, Clinique's Moisture Surge Overnight Mask will rehydrate parched skin.

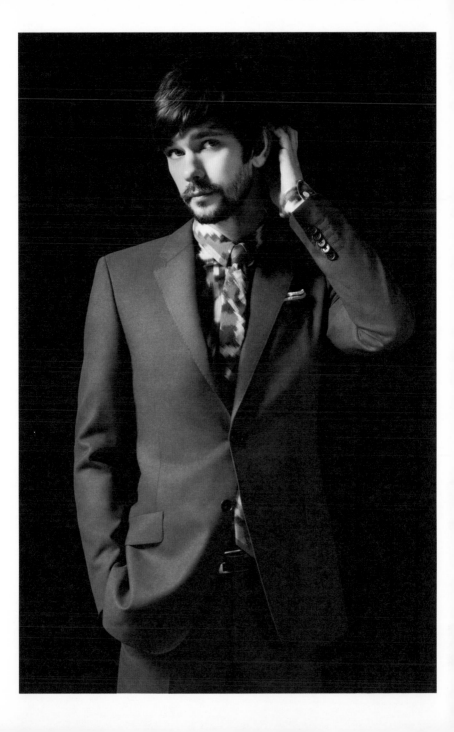

THE LOOK

MR BEN WHISHAW

From a lauded turn as Q in Skyfall *to his role in* Cloud Atlas, *the young British actor suits up and talks about breaking Hollywood*

Words by Mr Jonathan Heaf, features director of British *GQ*

THE FIRST TIME I spied Mr Ben Whishaw in the flesh – out in the real world, actual size, in original 3-D – was on the streets of Manhattan in 2010. The actor was, at the time, starring alongside Ms Andrea Riseborough – a rising talent herself – in an off-Broadway production of *The Pride*, written by playwright Mr Alexi Kaye Campbell and involving two parallel love stories between a man (Mr Hugh Dancy) and a woman (Ms Riseborough), and a man (Mr Dancy again) and another man (Mr Whishaw).

Looking half lost, half stoned and just a sprinkle self-conscious, Mr Whishaw shuffled apologetically past that day, eyes drilling down into the New York pavement in a manner that might be described as a little like Mr Kevin Spacey's cripple, Verbal, in *The Usual Suspects*. It seemed to me that Mr Whishaw was going to some pains to slope past unnoticed; happy to observe, rather than be observed. Still, I clocked him. Or thought I did. And prior to meeting him again three years later in a more official capacity I felt proud – no, sure – that this sighting confirmed all my assumed preconceptions of this most British of British actors: short, boyishly handsome, a little jumpy, a lot introverted, nice eyes and about as brazen and as bawdy as a newborn foal.

Of course, that's what everyone always thinks about Mr Whishaw: reluctant, fame-weary, bookish, and unfathomably thespian. Well, we're all spectacularly wrong. (Mostly wrong anyway; he is very thespian. And quite bookish.) And if his brilliantly erudite, assertive turn in the BBC's *The Hour* (as the wily Freddie Lyon) failed to convince you of such collective misreadings of the man, then his excellent reincarnation of James Bond's gadget guy, Q, in *Skyfall* in 2012 will have confirmed what you already suspected deep down: that there's more to this boy than meets the eye.

"I just keep myself to myself, mostly," says Mr Whishaw. "Perhaps that's why people don't see me as this larger-than-life... celebrity." To his credit, the way in which he almost retches out that last word like a cat coughing up a fur ball shows you his disregard – or rather, what little interest – he has in our cultural obsession with the famous for being famous.

"I do get stopped on the street, although rarely. And they always have something lovely to say. Someone was talking to me about that poor girl in the *Twilight* films – Kirsten, is it?"

Kristen.

"Kristen, that's right. I wouldn't like that. Not at all. Living in hotel rooms and being mobbed. A terrible state of existence. Terrible!"

Despite not enjoying the trappings of fame and glossing over the globe-spanning, box office-demolishing juggernaut that is the Bond franchise for just a second, 2013 turned out to be one of Mr Whishaw's most prolific years yet. First there was the Wachowskis' epic adaptation of Mr David Mitchell's purposefully rudderless *Cloud Atlas* – "I still don't know whether I understand all of it. Although I'm happy not to have every plot line sewn up neatly" – and then the Bedfordshire-born actor starred in *Peter and Alice* at the Noël Coward Theatre in London, alongside none other than M. That's right, his new, old boss, Dame Judi Dench.

"We actually never met on the set for Bond, Judi and I," says Mr Whishaw. "I think it was at the premiere that we first managed to say hello to one another properly. That whole Bond experience pretty much blew my mind – if only for my realisation of the insatiable global appetite for James Bond. His legacy will go on far longer than any of ours."

Still, there's no doubt of the admiration for Mr Whishaw, especially if Twitter is anything to go by. The morning I meet him, both the author Mr Bret Easton Ellis and journalist Ms Caitlin Moran tweet their lustful adorations of the good-natured boy-child – Ms Moran going so far as to say she'd like to "bang" him.

"I'm not aware of any of that stuff," he smiles, stifling a grin the size of a canoe. "But thank you for telling me. It's always nice to be appreciated."

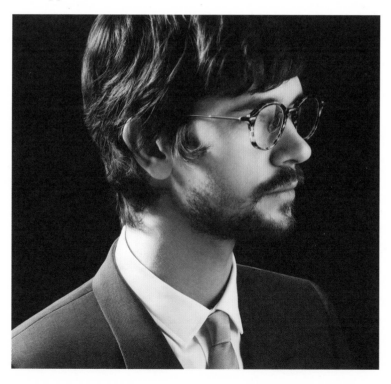

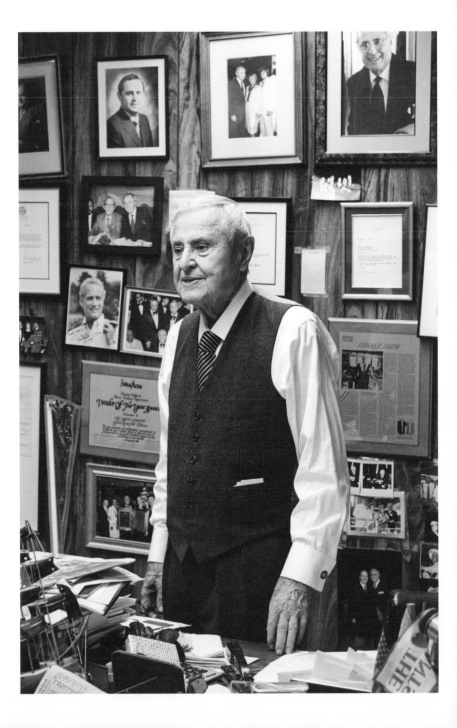

THE PRESIDENT'S TAILOR

*The man who has long dressed America's political elite,
Mr Martin Greenfield, has a life story that more than measures
up to any of his clients'*

Words by Mr Jeffrey Podolsky

I TOSS my light brown hacking coat with its velvet lapel over a chair and the legendary tailor Mr Martin Greenfield slowly gets up from behind his desk and softly says, "Let me hang your coat properly." I've travelled to Bushwick – a neighbourhood in Brooklyn not meant for the faint of heart – to meet Mr Greenfield and to learn a thing or two about tailoring and, as it turns out, life as well.

Then again, if such private customers as Messrs Paul Newman, Michael Jackson, Colin Powell, and three presidents (it has become common knowledge that President Barack Obama – in addition to former presidents Gerald Ford and Bill Clinton – is a client) have traipsed through this rough neighbourhood to meet Mr Greenfield, well so can I.

Mr Greenfield – dressed in a smart three-piece blue suit with a royal navy windowpane check, complemented by a narrow blue striped shirt and paisley tie (not to mention the Ronald Reagan presidential cufflinks given to him by Mr Powell, and a solid gold ring of the US dollar) – learnt his craft the hard way.

"You see, I love to dress up," Mr Greenfield says, in the ancient factory where he's worked (and later bought from his former employer) since he landed in the US in 1947, aged 19, and rose from floor boy to factory manager. "It shows you're important."

Mr Greenfield and his staff of approximately 125 cutters, sewers and pattern makers put together clothing for labels ranging from Brooks Brothers Golden Fleece to Band of Outsiders. His company, Martin Greenfield Clothiers, has produced made-to-order pieces for such brands as Donna Karan, Yves Saint Laurent and rag & bone.

But he revels in the art of the private client, which normally takes three fittings over eight weeks and whose prices begin at £1,650. "We measure correctly right from the beginning – poof, poof! – and it's right," Mr Greenfield says. "Other people fix here and there for these fittings. Not us."

Regardless of material, Mr Greenfield personally adores a crepe weave for suits. "It moves with you, and is the most comfortable to wear. Most men are colour-blind. You always need to know what a customer does for a living. Of course, the biggest bargain is quality – and the richest people tend to spend money the wrong way."

He's tended to the rich and famous of every stripe and size, whether it be the 7'1" basketball star Mr Shaquille O'Neal ("He needs a high rise. He's a big boy") to Mr Michael Jackson ("I met him when he just started as a baby. He was a very nice guy – then he died"). He holds a special affection for Mr Paul Newman – "a casual guy who initially favoured an old-fashioned sweat suit, but when we dressed him up, he loved his clothing" – and who once rang him up to announce he was retiring and putting all his tailor-made suits in a bonfire even though Mr Greenfield warned him otherwise. "He was something very special," recalls Mr Greenfield. "I said, 'You're still going to need those suits and return to the movies.'" Mr Greenfield, of course, proved correct.

The company produced the meticulously crafted prohibition-era outfits for the major characters of HBO's *Boardwalk Empire* and Mr Greenfield speaks fondly of lead actor Mr Steve Buscemi: "I asked him, 'What do you like best about the show?' He said, 'The clothing.'" As for Mr Ben Affleck and his critically acclaimed film *Argo*, Mr Greenfield laughs at where all the 1970s-era clothes, with their wide lapels and flares, ended up. "He kept all the suits and wears them!"

In the 1970s, when two secret servicemen bullied Mr Greenfield as they asked him to produce a couple of suits complete with custom-made bulletproof vests for then-president Gerald Ford, Mr Greenfield quickly reminded them: "I am a survivor and I don't let people push me around. So act like gentlemen and listen." And they did. Lest we forget this is a man who vividly remembers, upon arriving at Auschwitz (after first being showered, having his head shaved and his left arm tattooed), seeing the reflection of his face in Josef Mengele's shined boots as the infamous "Angel of Death" chose who would live or die then and there.

"I will meet you when we both survive," his father then told him. "We cannot be together because we're going to suffer for each other. You are strong."

"That was the last time I saw my family," says Mr Greenfield. "I never thought they would get buried or gassed. It was a sunny day in March."

His father proved right about his son, however: the young Mr Greenfield, a Czech by birth, outwitted his captors at every turn, whether at Auschwitz, during the infamous death marches, or at Buchenwald, where he recalls shaking hands as a little boy with General Dwight Eisenhower after US troops liberated the camp. "You could smell where the people were burned," he says.

In the end, says Mr Greenfield, "You learn how to respect people, how to do the right thing. The moment you become human again – you can live like a human being." Which he has clearly done – and doesn't plan to stop doing anytime soon. "I'll be here forever," says the man with the gentle voice, who's lived the most hardened of lives. "I'm not afraid to die because I never thought I would live long in those years I suffered through. But guess what: I'm here. And I thank God every day for that."

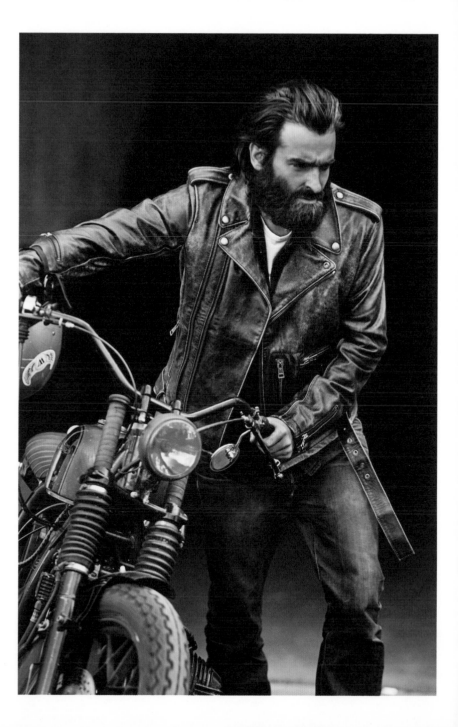

CUSTOM BIKE HEROES

MR PORTER meets two Parisians shaking up
the world of motorbike design

Words by Mr Mansel Fletcher, Features Editor, MR PORTER

I AM STANDING outside an anonymous multistorey car park in Paris' civilised but unremarkable 17th arrondissement. Venturing into the depths of the building, I discover a small space at the back that's part workshop, part hang-out. If grown men were able to create dens, the way that little boys do, then they'd look like this. There are vintage motorbikes and motorbike parts littering the floor. There's a ratty-looking sofa and a coffee table on which sit bourbon bottles. There's a nude calendar, and, tellingly, there's an iMac.

It's an undiluted dream of what a man's workspace should look like, and it is the home of Blitz Motorcycles, the custom bike shop run by Messrs Fred Jourden (who has a big beard) and Hugo Jezegabel (who has a smaller beard). It's here that they transform old motorbikes, from humble Japanese 125cc examples to grand vintage BMWs, into unique, individually tailored works of automotive art. Mr Jourden told MR PORTER about Blitz, while in the background Mr Jezegabel worked on the company's next project.

MR PORTER also learnt a valuable style lesson on the day of the interview: never wear a white shirt when visiting a garage.

Is your background mechanical?
I was an online marketing director when I started doing a night course in mechanics. When I was younger my father gave me lessons in engineering, so I knew how an engine worked but I had never put my hands inside one before. When I graduated I was the happiest man on earth.

How did Blitz begin?
After I graduated I worked with a friend who serviced bikes and we started to customise our first BMWs. Then one day the guy who owns this garage suggested I meet Hugo. I taught Hugo how to build a bike, and we built bikes for us, for friends and for friends of friends – all for free. Then in 2009 the financial crisis came and I took it as a sign; Blitz was formed in 2010.

What kind of bikes do you customise?
We don't have a specific brand focus. We have worked on BMW, Harley-Davidson, Yamaha, Kawasaki, Honda, Triumph and Royal Enfield. However, we never work on fuel-injected bikes because to change the tank we have to reinstall a fuel pump and they will go wrong. So we only do bikes with carburettors.

What is the Blitz aesthetic?
We love imperfection. We love to mix shiny paint with rust, dents and scratches. It's like a scuffed vintage leather jacket; I want the jacket to tell a story. We're trying to give a bit of soul to the bike.

What does it mean that you tailor the bikes for the client?
There's a bike we made on the base of a Kawasaki 650 for a guy who runs a company called Jawa Productions. We knew, but he didn't, that there is a Czech bike brand called Jawa. So we fitted a Jawa tank, added a bit of dust, a bit of rust, some chrome and some burgundy paint and told him, this is your Jawasaki. Another client is an English guy from Birmingham who's a gentleman and a punk

rocker. He said, "I want something posh and chic." But we know him and he's not always posh and chic; sometimes he's a bit dirty. So we went for a BSA tank, a bit of chrome, a bit of black, a bit of dust and a bit of rust. We called it a BSW and when he saw it he was happy.

Can you explain the appeal of your bikes, when they're so slow compared with sports bikes?
We make machines that you can control from your hips so you can enjoy a curve at 90kph and you have the feeling of surfing on the road. Cruising smoothly on secondary roads is best, because you can smell the forest and the flowers; if you see a river you can stop and have a swim – it's like being a cowboy. Also, there's a big speed repression in France – you can't go faster than 50kph in the city.

Did you set out to appeal to guys who don't feel part of the conventional bike community?
We'd rather have a little coverage in a fashion magazine, a design magazine or a women's magazine than in a bike magazine. We're trying to pull the bike out of its redneck world of bad taste, to bring it to something more edgy and beautiful. If we were to make a wish it would be to exhibit a bike at MoMA.

How have the bike manufacturers reacted?
BMW is supporting us, showing our films on its website and we have a bike in the BMW museum in Munich, even though it has a Yamaha tank. The other brands know we exist, but they don't need us. Triumph is already cool and Harley-Davidson is cool to a lot of people.

How did you come to work with Edwin?
The marketing manager asked if he could work with us after he saw our film *Riding September*. First we built a bike for Edwin, and while we built it we exchanged long emails about the philosophy of life, and we ended up working on a capsule collection.

What constitutes the Blitz look?
A jumper from Saint James, a T-shirt from Edwin, a pair of Edwin jeans, Red Wing boots, a vintage watch and a vintage leather jacket, or in summer an antique Belstaff jacket. And we go for Davida helmets, which have the look of the 1960s.

Who are your biking heroes?
Bud Ekins, Steve McQueen's friend. He was a stunt rider who made the jump on *The Great Escape* because the studio wouldn't let McQueen do it. Evel Knievel, because he made me dream as a kid; Giacomo Agostini; and Barry Sheene, of course.

What kind of bike would you most like to work on?
The dream bike would be a Vincent Black Lightning. It's a famous English brand, wonderfully done, but respected too much. I'd like to put a Yamaha tank on it, but it will never happen as those bikes are so rare and when we strip a bike down there's no way back.

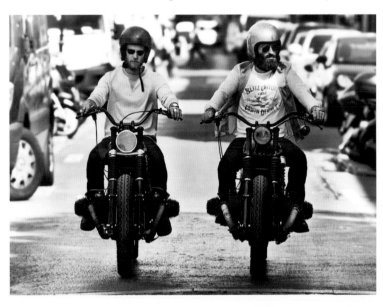

THE REPORT

MR PABLO PICASSO

*We pay tribute to the man whose style was
as inspirational as his art*

Words by Dr Michael Peppiatt, author, critic and art historian

WERE THEY bright red, breaking on two-tone shoes, or criss-crossed in loud golfer's check? Were they unexpectedly formal, hind parts of a bespoke suit, or baggy plus fours with Argyle socks? Were they ever tuxedo trousers before they metamorphosed into summer slacks or shrank into jaunty pre-war Riviera swimsuits?

They were all of these and many more, since Mr Pablo Picasso changed the way he dressed as often and as radically as he changed the way he painted. He was as instinctive a dresser as he was an artist, replacing one look with another every time something in his life or his fantasy prompted it. Many of the artists around him dressed quite conventionally, above all when success caught up with them. There was Mr Georges Braque in his cool white scarf, Mr Henri Matisse plumply avuncular in a waistcoat while sketching a nude, or Mr Wassily Kandinsky as formally attired as an old-school banker. Mr Salvador Dalí, it's true, put on a show, with the twirled mustachios, the fur coats and silver-topped canes. But Mr Picasso wasn't putting on a show. Whether dressed for the opera, disguised for a *bal masqué* or simply clowning about, he was always himself – or one of his many selves.

"Only superficial people do not judge by appearances," said Mr Oscar Wilde – bless him! And I look forward to one day reading some learned thesis on how artists present themselves to the world and why. Mr Francis Bacon dressed in later life like a successful gangster, an upper-class, English Al Capone in tight, perfectly cut double-breasted suits with subtle stripes and threatening black leather coats, also tight, with epaulettes. Frivolous? I'm not sure. Everything he wore had its meaning for Mr Bacon, and you can even find the clothes he loved – particularly rainbow-hued silk shirts and desert boots – in his pictures. Is it merely anecdotal that Mr Alberto Giacometti invariably worked in a tweed jacket and tie, however caked in plaster, paint and clay they became? I don't think so. Challenging accepted vision every day in his Montparnasse hovel, Mr Giacometti clung to whatever shreds or threads of normality he could find.

The last time I bumped into Mr David Hockney, he had just stepped out of his West End tailors. They were making him a new suit, he explained amiably, and the scales fell from my eyes. That instantly recognisable look Mr Hockney had crafted over the years, from bright caps and stripy shirts to odd socks and comfortably baggy suits, was part of a carefully orchestrated show, mirroring his unstoppable rise from pop art icon to cultural grandee.

Style, they say, is the man. So how did Mr Picasso, the master artificer of the 20th century, choose to project himself? Did he limit himself to this look or that? Did he decide at a certain point to wear his trousers wide with a crease so sharp (like his friend, the poet Mr Jean Cocteau) that they could cut a Camembert in half? Of course not. He was a creature of infinite fantasy and infinite change. And having just looked through a few scores of photos of the *maître* at different moments in his long career, I can attest that he virtually never appeared before the camera in the same garb twice. Catch him if you can. During his early years in Paris he would be in vaguely artisanal dress, dark overalls and donkey jackets, occasionally spruced up by a broad-brimmed hat or Romantic *lavallière*. Then without warning he appears in clunky gaiters or, bizarrely, in an army uniform he had borrowed from

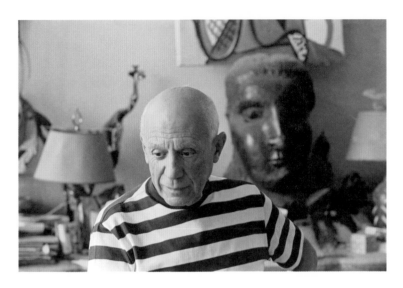

Mr Picasso at Villa La Californie, Cannes, France, 1957

his co-cubist, Mr Braque. These were early days, but it was already clear that Mr Picasso enjoyed not just dressing but dressing up.

At this point Mr Picasso was still seeking recognition. But as he outraged then entranced the rich by his challenging imagery, he transformed his own appearance from dangerous iconoclast to cuddly lounge lizard. Out went any trace of dungaree and sweater and in came the perfect suit and tie, hatted and hankied, with just a hint of a waistcoat and a cuff-linked sleeve. This was Mr Picasso's so-called "Duchess" period, when all the aristocratic and moneyed doors opened to him and he, totally self-aware and totally self-promotional, dressed for his new role in life.

But once he proved his ability to look – more or less – like the nobs who paid high prices for his pictures, he realised he no longer needed to reassure them. After all he was now sufficiently wealthy and well established to lounge at the back of his chauffeured Hispano-Suiza in his underwear if he cared to. "I want to be rich enough," he once declared, "to live like someone who's poor." To him that meant messing around freely and eating in shorts in the kitchen and not giving a toss if an important dealer or collector dropped by. In a trice he went happily from top hat to beret and espadrilles, from three-piece to no-piece (or almost), since his life was now focused either on the studio, the bed or the beach.

Even so, the love of dressing up remained. Mr Picasso always found something to clown around in before the camera, whether it was a huge false nose, a lugubrious deerstalker or the magnificent Indian headdress Mr Gary Cooper had given him. As Mr Picasso grew older he wore less and less, often sporting no more than a Mediterranean tan and swimming trunks. But by then he was the most famous and most photographed artist in the world, and so instantly recognisable he no longer really needed clothes.

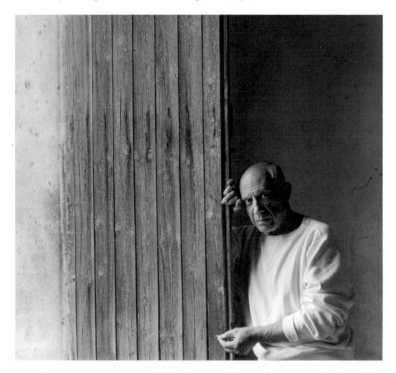

Mr Picasso in Vallauris, France, 1954

CUTTING-EDGE LIVING

Nine intriguing designs from the world's
greatest furniture fair

Words by Mr Nick Vinson

MILAN'S SALONE DEL MOBILE is arguably the most important date on the global design calendar. Each April, the great and the good of the design world – leading architects, industrial and interior designers, buyers, curators, gallerists and journalists – descend on Milan en masse. In 2013, more than 324,000 jetted in from all over the world – from more than 160 countries no less – to take in as many new sofas, chairs, tables, bookshelves and lamps as they could in a packed six days.

Aside from the official fairgrounds where the leading Italian and international furniture brands present works, every possible space in the city is taken over to exhibit what is new in furniture and design. Alongside brands that prefer to exhibit in their own showrooms, there are those that choose to rent some jewel-like locations normally hidden from the public.

Then there are the fashion houses presenting their lucrative home collections and unveiling design collaborations, such as Versace Home with The Haas Brothers, Missoni's store by design darling Ms Patricia Urquiola, Bottega Veneta's one-of-a-kind boxes with artist Ms Nancy Lorenz, and Prada, which hosted the launch of the week: on the very same set used for its fall/winter show, the architect Mr Rem Koolhaas of the Office for Metropolitan

Architecture launched Tools for Life, the much-anticipated first line of furniture for renowned American maker Knoll. Visiting from Paris was Hermès, with eight new furniture pieces by Mr Philippe Nigro, and Louis Vuitton, which hosted a series of design talks with the top talent behind its Objets Nomades line.

During the fair, days are spent pounding the *padiglioni* (or halls of the fairgrounds) and evenings spent passing from one venue to the next, *aperitivo* in hand. The design calendar is packed with openings, parties and tempting dinners, however it's in Milan where you learn to just sip and nibble, as you can be expected to dine three times in one night. Here are the designs that impressed us the most...

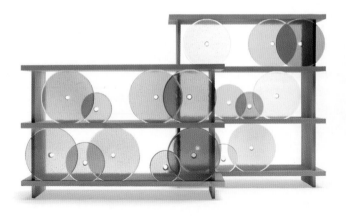

ROTATING GLASS SHELF
By Nendo for Dilmos

In 2003, the Japanese design office of Nendo, headed by Mr Oki Sato, made its debut at Salone Satellite, the part of Salone del Mobile where young talents hope to get noticed by manufacturers. Nendo certainly did. Fast forward to 2013 and it presented products for 15 different brands and had no less than four different exhibitions, one of which was *Glassworks* at Dilmos gallery. It was borderline overkill, yet Nendo's poetic design is so good that you can almost forgive the company. This shelf, in birch wood with glass disks made by leading glass and lighting specialist Lasvit, owes something to Ms Charlotte Perriand's 1950s Mexique bookshelf. Here, the finger-sized holes in the softly coloured disks become handles so that they can be easily rotated and repositioned.

THE IC LIGHTS SERIES
By Michael Anastassiades
for Flos

A signature of the London-based, Cypriot-born designer Mr Michael Anastassiades is his sublime lighting. For Euroluce 2013, Salone del Mobile's biannual lighting fair, he teamed up with Flos, one of Italy's most prestigious and technically advanced lighting producers. The pairing did not disappoint; Mr Anastassiades' String suspension lights cleverly integrated the normally problematic cable issue into the design. And he delighted with the IC Lights series, shown here, as seemingly unstable glass spheres magically balance on anthracite or brushed brass stems. A delicate equilibrium fit for a juggler.

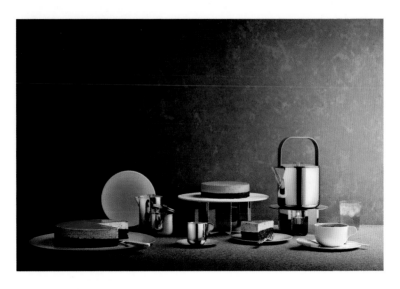

TEA WITH GEORG TEA SET
By Scholten & Baijings for Georg Jensen

Amsterdam-based Scholten & Baijings marries traditional craft and industrial production with an original use of colour. Tea with Georg is Mr Stefan Scholten and Ms Carole Baijings' first collaboration with Copenhagen-based silversmith Georg Jensen. This new tea set includes a teapot with warmer, a cake stand, and cups and saucers for both tea and espresso. The innovative use of materials, in this case stainless steel – a Jensen trademark – and Japanese porcelain and acrylic, is typical of Scholten & Baijings.

CONSOLE, TABLE AND CHAIR
By David Collins for Promemoria

The London-based architect-designer Mr David Collins was the man behind many a famous hotel, bar and restaurant – think London's The Wolseley, J Sheekey, The Delaunay, Claridge's Bar and The Blue Bar at the Berkeley. However, there was much more to Mr Collins than cocktails and fine dining, as his redesign for

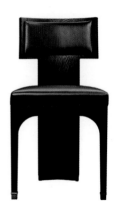

the Alexander McQueen stores proved, as did this capsule collection for furniture maker Promemoria. Tragically, Mr Collins died, all too young, in 2013, but this, the only commercially available range he produced, was shown in Milan before his passing. And a fitting tribute it is too.

LE PARC
By Rodolfo Dordoni for Minotti

Milan-based architect and designer Mr Rodolfo Dordoni, the go-to guy for contemporary with a hint of retro, coordinates and designs for Minotti, the Italian contemporary furniture powerhouse. Le Parc, the indoor/outdoor collection, was inspired by traditional European wrought-iron furniture, yet – and this is always Mr Dordoni's supreme skill – it has none of the normally characteristic frills. Instead, his is a correct and contemporary update; Le Parc includes sofas, armchairs, ottomans, benches, tables and a chaise longue, all in curved tubular iron covered in water-resistant upholstery.

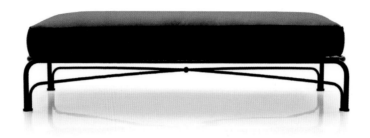

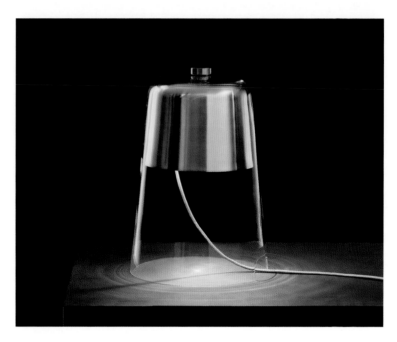

SEMPLICE LAMP
By Industrial Facility for Oluce

For his first lamp for storied maker Oluce, London-based industrial designer Mr Sam Hecht of Industrial Facility has eliminated both the base and the stem so that the glass rests directly on the table. The dimmer on the top holds the glass bell together with the spun metal canopy, seemingly containing the light source. These are all very deliberate reductions, and this is why Mr Hecht called this lamp Semplice, meaning "simple" in Italian.

EARTHQUAKE 5.9 VASE
By Patricia Urquiola for Budri

When an earthquake with a magnitude of 5.9 struck the Italian region of Emilia in May 2012, Budri, the Mirandola-based marble inlay atelier, was not spared the force of its violence, with its store of marble and semi-precious stones receiving a major hammering. Upon hearing the news, Milan-based designer Ms Patricia Urquiola teamed up with the company on a project using the quake-damaged slabs. The results were shown during Salone del Mobile 2013, and included bookcases, tables and striped triangular vases, one of which is shown here.

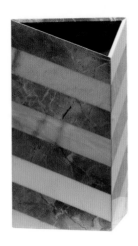

JUST BLACK
By Marsotto edizioni

The family-run firm Marsotto has been shaping marble for more than 150 years. In 2009, with the design help of the brilliant Milan-based Brit (and now sadly late) Mr James Irvine, it introduced Marsotto edizioni, a collection of furniture crafted from Marsotto's own marble. Other notable designers who contributed to the project include Munich's Mr Konstantin Grcic, Tokyo's Mr Naoto Fukasawa and London's Mr Jasper Morrison. Until now each piece was shown in white Carrara marble; the "just black" Marquina marble gives a totally new look and feel to the collection.

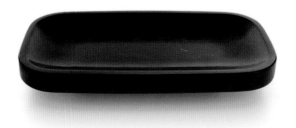

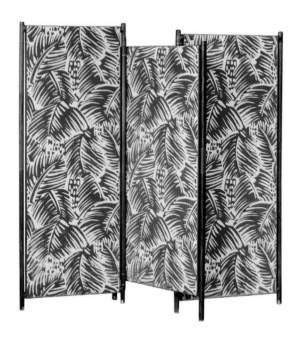

LES NÉCESSAIRES D'HERMÈS
By Philippe Nigro

Les Nécessaires d'Hermès is a collection of furniture designed with grooming and dressing in mind. The eight pieces have been designed by Mr Philippe Nigro, a French-born designer based in Milan who has the honour of not only working with Hermès but having his work sit beside that of masters including Mr Jean-Michel Frank, Mr Enzo Mari and Ms Rena Dumas. Crafted from materials including Canaletto walnut wood and Hermès bull calf leather, the partition, grooming unit (replete with rotating mirror and accessory compartments) and coat rack and accessory holder are all designed to take care of your fineries while you dress and undress.

THE GEAR

DESK LAMPS

*10 icons of engineering that deserve
a place in any man's work space*

Words by Mr Nick Compton

THE DESK LAMP is one of design's favourite problems. It has obsessed engineers who should have been busy with other things and driven them to decades of distraction. The British engineer Mr George Carwardine came up with the now iconic Anglepoise in the 1930s. It was the game-changer. Now you could alter a light's height, direction and position with a touch rather than through a tiresome process of unclamping, twisting and turning. It has been endlessly imitated, generating a whole new typology.

Mr Richard Sapper's Tizio is a sort of masterpiece, a study in balance and beautifully realised functionality. And though it was designed in the early 1970s, it gained totemic momentum in the 1980s and became the altar-piece in the mat-black dream home. Other designers have placed formal elegance before flexibility and functionality, putting together sometimes stark, sometimes delicate compositions of shape, material and light.

More attention is now being paid to quality of light – computer screens present different lighting challenges to ink on paper – and energy efficiency. The major Italian lighting brands such as Flos and Artemide are using LEDs to produce lamps that give off a kinder, gentler light and are kinder and gentler to the planet. Here are 10 lamps that would look at home on the desk of any man of influence.

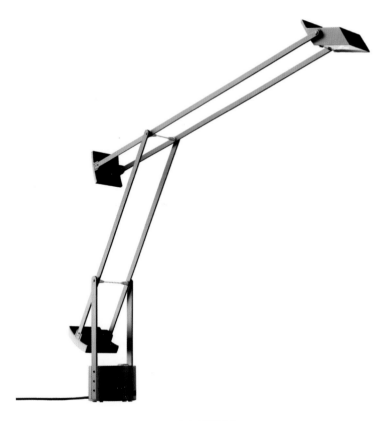

THE TIZIO

Designed by German Mr Richard Sapper in 1972, the Tizio is as radical an innovation and as elegant a design solution as the Anglepoise. Two delicately counterbalanced arms allow for the most graceful of movement while the parallel arms conduct electricity, keeping the design free of trailing wires. The use of a halogen bulb was also a novelty at the time (one downside was that the bulb got very hot so a thin wire handle was added to the head in the 1990s). Though designed in the 1970s, the Tizio was way ahead of its time and really found commercial and critical favour – and became hugely influential – in the 1980s.

THE SNOOPY

Despite the jokey tag, the Snoopy is a cast-iron – or rather white marble and enamelled aluminium – classic 20th-century design. Launched in 1967, it was the work of the legendary Castiglioni brothers, Messrs Achille and Pier Giacomo. The appeal of the lamp lies in its marvellous match of material, colour and form and an underlying tension in the design. Snoopy looks as if it should topple backwards, the elegant marble base not up to supporting the reflector, but a heavy glass disc acts as a counterweight to keep the lamp magically upright.

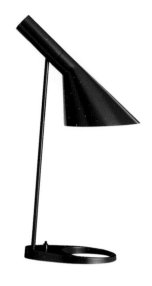

THE AJ

The "AJ" stands for design legend Mr Arne Jacobsen, who designed this lamp (as well as the now ubiquitous Swan and Egg chairs) for the SAS Royal Hotel in Copenhagen in 1960. Mr Jacobsen was a master of strong, simple shapes and striking profiles and the AJ, with its moveable, slightly sinister hood, is instantly recognisable. The cut-out in the cast-iron base was originally designed to hold an ashtray but welcomes other applications. The lamp is now available in a range of colours.

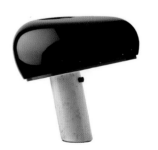

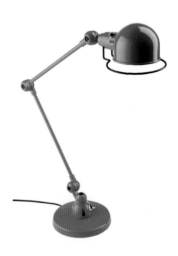

THE BINIC

Named after a lighthouse on the coast of Brittany, the Binic has a pleasantly briny air about it, recalling the brightly coloured cowl vents on boats (though from other angles it looks oddly like the permanently imperilled Kenny from *South Park*). The work of the Breton designer Ms Ionna Vautrin, this playful, and at just 8" tall, dinky little lamp has an aluminium base and a polycarbonate head and comes in a range of colours.

THE SIGNAL

If the Anglepoise is the iconic British task light, the French favour the similar, and similarly flexible, Signal, produced in Lyon since 1953. And like the Anglepoise, the Signal was the work of an inventive engineer rather than a designer. Mr Jean-Louis Domecq spent a decade developing the design before establishing a company, Jieldé, to produce it. Made in a number of different colours in enamelled steel, the Signal lamp is an enduring piece of industrial funk.

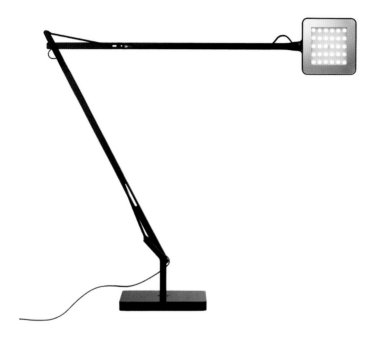

THE KELVIN

The Kelvin is Mr Antonio Citterio's hi-tech, energy-efficient and impossibly elegant take on the post-Anglepoise typology. The load-compensating spring is housed inside the lamp's aluminium arms while 30 LEDs are combined to produce a soft, diffused light. A "green" sensor can also be activated by simply swiping your hand across the lamp head. The Kelvin will then adjust its output to match the room's ambient light, saving on energy use. You can also use the ariel swipe method to turn the light off.

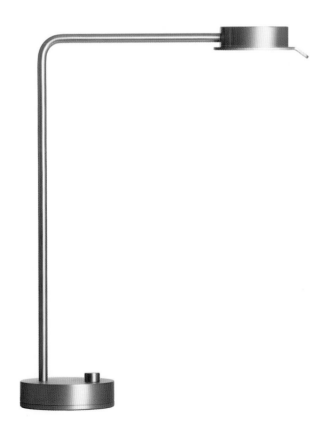

THE CHIPPERFIELD WIO2

Named after its designer, British architect Sir David Chipperfield, this is a minimalist's delight, a single joint-free line drawn in brass connecting two simple discs. And while the Chipperfield has an air of rugged rigidity, ball-bearings in the base actually make for smooth-running rotation. A rubber base means the lamp is more surface friendly than it might first appear while the rotatable head houses dimmable LED bulbs.

THE PIANI

Designed by the French fraternal design duo, Messrs Ronan and Erwan Bouroullec, the Piani is all about the tray at the base of the lamp, which the pair sees as a sort of spotlit stage for small objects. Masters of material and minimal forms, the duo's Piani is a high-gloss but clean-lined instant classic and comes in plastic and oak and in a range of colours.

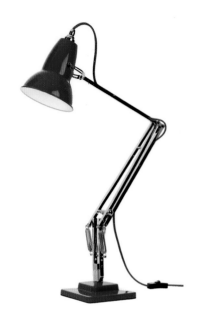

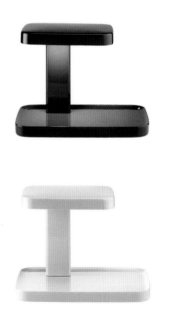

THE ANGLEPOISE 1227

Initially launched in 1934, Mr Carwardine's Anglepoise 1227 lamp is a genuine British design icon, a triumph of elegant engineering and up-front functionality. The Anglepoise 1227 used three springs to hold its arms in place without the need for clamps, while its Art-Deco base added dramatic support. The design has been updated various times and Sir Kenneth Grange's Type 75, launched in 2004, is a minimalist masterwork in its own right.

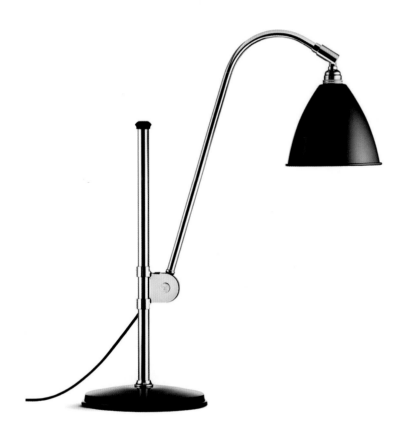

THE BESTLITE BLI

Another great British design, though with a strong Bauhaus influence, the Bestlite was the work of British designer Mr Robert Dudley Best, who studied in Paris and Düsseldorf. It has been produced by the family firm in Birmingham since 1930 (at that time, the world's largest lighting factory). Though still made in Birmingham, the manufacturing rights were taken over by Danish company Gubi in 2004, which upped the quality and gave the design a new lease of life. Gubi also produces another classic of Bauhaus-influenced modernism, Ms Greta Grossman's Cobra lamp.

MR JAKE BUGG

*The British singer-songwriter shares
his five favourite tracks*

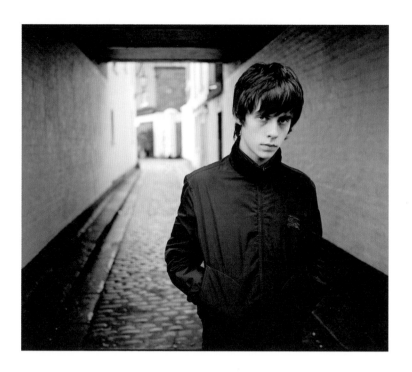

"Leave My Woman Alone"
RAY CHARLES

"It's got a consistent feel to it and a really cool vibe."

"I Don't Wanna Know"
JOHN MARTYN

"It's a really nice track that's quite mellow. It's got a bit of a jazz instrumental in the middle section, but the actual song is well structured."

"Twilight Time"
THE PLATTERS

"There's a lot of melodic changes in this one. I didn't like it when I first heard it – but it's one of those songs where the more you listen, the more you get from it."

"Alone Again Or"
LOVE

"I love the story behind this – if it's true, that is. Apparently they were criminals on the run and they'd hold up stores, but they made beautiful music. This track's great."

"Use Me"
BILL WITHERS

"I love those off-beat drums man – it's f***ing great."

ALFRESCO DINING PERKS
(AND PERILS)

Why eating outdoors isn't always
such a bright idea...

Words by Mr Dan Davies and Ms Sophie Dening

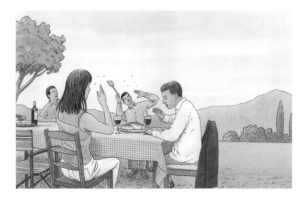

EATING OUTDOORS is idealised, not least by those of us whose lives are spent cowering under pregnant, slate-grey skies (and that's only when summer really gets into its stride). Dining alfresco conjures quintessential images of the Mediterranean: weathered tables, artfully mismatched chairs, gingham tablecloths and bottles of wine replenished by waiters working via telepathy. Blue skies, the sun on your skin and lazy afternoons that turn into pleasantly drunken evenings. Good times.

Or not. Whatever experts say about the science of food tasting better in the great outdoors or the psychological benefits of feeling closer to nature, there are pitfalls awaiting the northern European who remains determined to follow the lead of his southern cousins.

Let us begin with nature, as we seem to become preoccupied with it once the sun comes out. In case you hadn't noticed, humans are not alone among God's children in enjoying the warm weather. Insects live for it, and their attitude seems to be that if we're eating outside, then they'll invite themselves along too. Just look across the terrace or garden at the diner waving their arms around in a manner that suggests they're attempting to park a particularly large plane in a hurry.

Then, when the weather gets really warm, there are the additional delights of mosquitoes. Do you protect yourself with socks and endure the sensation of your feet squelching in sweat, swathe yourself in so much insect repellent that your eyes water, or spend the meal scratching furiously at the freshly sucked welts around your ankles? No, you just take the sensible option and eat inside.

Further up the food chain, things don't get much better. Anyone who has tried eating fish and chips out of the paper in a British seaside town will testify to the perils of seagulls swooping out of the skies like demented extras from *Jurassic Park*. In cities, it's their witless relations, the pigeons, with their dollops of avian mayonnaise delivered with unerring accuracy from on high. When it comes to dining, my view is that birds should either be chirping from distant trees or served up on a plate.

Dogs have no place at the table either, and yet they have become a fixture in the gardens of so-called "dog-friendly" gastro pubs. Tell me what's so friendly about catching sight of a random canine meticulously lapping at its nether region when you're about to take a mouthful of over-priced food? The same goes for "child-friendly" outdoor eating spaces, unless of course your idea of a relaxing meal is the cacophonous backdrop of kids crying, falling over, hitting each other, being stung by wasps or admonished by flustered parents for picking bits of food off the floor that have presumably been left behind by the flies, pigeons and dogs.

Of course, dining alfresco is all about the weather but there are too many permutations to make it anything but a precarious experience. If it's too hot and you're in the wrong chair, you'll sweat through your shirt and be heading home with sunburn that is reminiscent of Mr David Bowie's Aladdin Sane character; if you're in the shade, what are you doing eating outside in the first place? Forget your sunglasses and you'll spend the meal squinting like a daytime drunk (however much or little you've had to drink); wear them and you won't be able to properly appreciate the food on the plate before you. If the wind gets up you'll be contending with waves in your gazpacho; if it rains – or if you're in the UK, *when* it rains – you'll be cursing yourself for being so stupid.

If only every terrace offered the bucolic charm and tranquillity of the one at the late El Bulli on the Costa Brava. The reality, however, is rather different. The desire to eat under the sun or the stars means that we all too often pretend away the drone of passing traffic, passenger jets or the incessant rattling of the air-conditioning unit positioned conveniently above your head. Diners wouldn't be expected to put up with such noise pollution inside a restaurant, so why do we become so tolerant when outside?

Then there is the paranoia, a by-product of the devil-may-care attitude many exhibit when consuming their dinner in the great outdoors. If you're seated at a table on the street in a big city, and you're anything like me, you'll be concentrating less on the menu than on patting the pocket of your trousers to ensure that your iPhone and wallet haven't been hoisted. That and reminding your wife or date that she really shouldn't leave her handbag gaping like an open invitation to passing pickpockets. Both have the net result of rather killing the romance of the setting (unless, of course, you're sitting directly underneath the air-conditioning unit, from where she won't be able to hear what you're saying anyway).

To cap it all off, you're destined to spend most of your outside time waving at the waiter to try to get his attention. The problem is, he will almost certainly think you are being attacked by a wasp, fending off the attentions of a particularly hungry pigeon or throwing your hands up in despair at the fact that your toddler has just had his first course from the wheelie bins. Good luck with it all. I'll be eating inside, watching it all through an open window.

SIX OPEN-AIR SPOTS THAT CAN'T BE SPOILT

L'AVANT-PORT
Île de Ré, France

L'Avant Port's elite location on the far side of St Martin's little quay, near the yacht club and away from the ice-cream kiosks, means very few passers-by, even in this most swarming of Île de Ré's pretty towns. Come for classic harbour views, discreet service and a daily catch of grilled prawns or roast langoustine tails.

CASA OAXACA
Oaxaca City, Mexico

In the spectacular city of Oaxaca, built in a valley on a plateau 5,000ft above sea level, gourmet pilgrims usually find their way to the mountain-view rooftop dining room at Casa Oaxaca. Authentic Mexican dishes are served – tacos, tostadas – but at a super-refined level, with seriously fine local produce.

CATALINA ROSE BAY
Sydney, Australia

This sleek restaurant on Sydney Harbour's eastern shore is open all day, serving oysters shucked to order, house-smoked salmon, roasted suckling pig and great pan-fried fish. The views from the terrace are fantastic: this is where the old flying boats used to take off for Southampton in the 1930s and 1940s.

HÔTEL AMERICANO
New York City, US

Cool rooftop dining near the High Line in Chelsea? Yes, please. Start with lobster, quinoa and avocado, then go for grilled New York strip steak with *chimichurri*. The brunch menu features super-berry açai smoothies and home-made granola. This was the first US project from Mexico's Grupo Habita, and the interior design is by MCH Arnaud Montigny, which also did the Colette store in Paris.

LOCANDA ANTICA MONTIN
Venice, Italy

A charming, old-fashioned *pensione* with iron beds and marble floors, and a gem of a restaurant in an open courtyard. The Venetian cuisine is anything but sophisticated, and you'll drink humble local wines, but the setting is magical. It's a favourite of restaurateur Mr Russell Norman, who says: "No matter how busy the city may be outside, it is always quiet and serene."

RIVER CAFÉ
London, UK

Still one of the best London restaurants, the River Café is a treat no matter what the weather; but on a sunny day, in the right company, there's nothing to beat sitting at one of its white-naped Thames-side tables, sipping something *frizzante* and looking forward to wood-roasted Scottish langoustines, chargrilled wild sea bass or Ligurian fish stew.

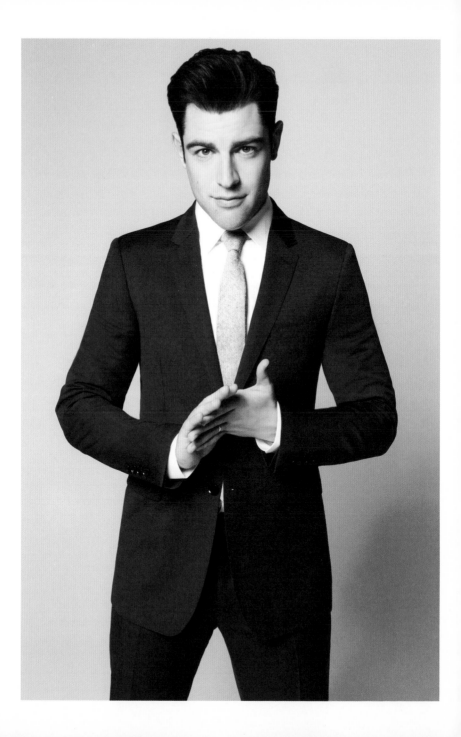

MR MAX GREENFIELD

The actor behind Schmidt in New Girl
talks viral videos and vanity

Words by Mr Jonathan Hey

AFTER the international success of Fox's sitcom *New Girl*, Mr Max Greenfield has become something of a comedy icon. That's because his character, Schmidt, is such a ridiculous, over-the-top, self-important, loveable loser – a perfect foil to the wide-eyed optimism of his roommate Jess, played so indelibly by Ms Zooey Deschanel.

As Schmidt's popularity has risen, thanks, in part, to several viral videos Mr Greenfield made, including one of Schmidt's dating profile (his perfect match? Himself) and another where he teaches a spinning class to an empty room with the energy of a banshee, so has his red carpet quotient.

In 2013, after swooning over a certain designer in a guest-edited entry for Ms Gwyneth Paltrow's website, Goop (the actress tweeted about how big a fan she was of his character), Mr Greenfield finally got his wish: the designer sent him a tuxedo to wear at the Golden Globes, for which Mr Greenfield was nominated for his role in *New Girl*.

"I will never own a nicer piece of clothing in all of my life," says Mr Greenfield, who grew up in Westchester, New York, and now lives in Los Angeles with his wife, Ms Tess Sanchez, a casting director, and their daughter, Lilly. "You feel like a different man.

That thing fits you in a way that you think – maybe I could kick some ass in this thing. Sometimes I just wear it around the house. I'm not proud of it, but every once in a while I'll just put it on and say, 'Honey, take a look at me in this thing'."

You've done an incredible job of making Schmidt "live" off television screens. Was that always on the cards?
Well, that's what we wanted to do. We've turned it into a kind of performance piece. I fully understand the joke of Schmidt and I had some outside ideas I wanted to play with. That's how the spinning class video happened. It was, "Look, I know where I live on this, and what my position is, and if it continues to gain momentum and success I'm going to be Kramer from *Seinfeld*." Definitely of my co-stars, my character is certainly the most showy. Rather than going, "No I'm not like him", or "I'm not going to do that", I fully embraced it. I said, "Let's go at it 100%." The idea is to let people know that you are so in on the joke that you maybe supersede the pigeonhole of it all.

Did you know the viral videos would find an audience?
The online dating profile making fun of *The Hills* – that I knew was a home run. The spin video I did not. That one was just fun. *New York Magazine*'s Vulture website had written a piece on Schmidt's work-out ethic, and I said, "I will show you exactly what it looks like", and we went and shot it. And then we put it up and people freaked out. You have to find these little pockets of interest. And you can really hit hard in that one place of the 18% that go, "Yes, you did that correctly". And there's another 82% going, "What is this?".

Have any celebrities asked you for advice on how to go viral?
No. It's no secret that you've just got to find the right concept. You've got to know how to get out on the internet and catch or impact the right audience. As for Twitter, you can't overthink it. It's all

about content and getting stuff out there and letting people know what you're doing. Lena Dunham is great at it. Mindy Kaling is great at it. It's really important to create a personality on Twitter, so that whomever reads your feed doesn't just read it, they hear you saying it.

Has playing Schmidt changed the way you dress?
Well I've got some nice clothing. I do like to dress it up a little. It's fun. I like my clothes. I like to pick out stuff myself. I'm a big fan of Band of Outsiders. I've always loved them. I love the Black Fleece by Brooks Brothers stuff by Thom Browne. And it's fun to put on a Gucci suit and do a photoshoot and think, "Man, I feel slick right now." And then when I got dressed for the Golden Globes I was like, "I'm in the James Bond suit."

What would Schmidt's 10 style commandments be?
I feel as if any rules he creates are solely based on what time it is. They're ever changing. He's just a guy who opens up a magazine, sees Justin Timberlake in a suit and tries to carry that off as his own, as if he's never seen it. I think probably to some degree that could sum it up, because Justin Timberlake is maybe the furthest thing away from a chubby Jewish kid who is really uncomfortable in his own skin.

Is there anything Mr Timberlake has done that Schmidt would not?
Not a thing. He definitely would have been into the denim phase. He would have watched that HBO concert and said, "There it is. That defines how I want to live my life and how I want to be perceived." But Schmidt's spins are horrible and totally ruin it. Everywhere Justin Timberlake goes right, Schmidt goes wrong.

Does Schmidt like fancy sneakers?
Yeah, he likes fancy everything.

What is your philosophy about shoes?
All you need is a good pair of boots and a nice pair of dress shoes.
I'm not big on wearing sneakers. I like to wear them for a work-
out. I've never been that guy, but if you rock a pair of Converse
I'm totally into it.

Is there anything you always travel with?
I'm really into a V neck, like this Black Fleece one I'm wearing.
I take this pretty much everywhere. It's always good to have it. You
can dress it up a little, you can throw it over a T-shirt. It's a nice,
kind-of-covers-everything item. If I had a uniform it would be
a blue V-neck sweater.

What else have you enjoyed working on?
I did a movie called *They Came Together* in 2012. It's by David Wain
and Michael Showalter, kind of like a *Wet Hot American Summer*
2. If they invited me to do a movie every summer, I would take no
money and show up wherever they wanted me. And the cast was
just insane: Paul Rudd and Amy Poehler and all the guys from
The State. These people are on another level.

Would you ever consider doing a Schmidt clothing line?
No.

ART-DECO DRIVES

The cars that put the "roar" into the
"Roaring Twenties" and beyond

Words by Mr Tom M Ford, Features Writer, MR PORTER

IN 2013, the Frist Center for the Visual Arts in Nashville presented *Sensuous Steel: Art Deco Automobiles*. It was the first major exhibition of its kind, for which 18 unique cars were painstakingly sourced by Virginia-based curator Mr Ken Gross for their history, style and sheer Art-Deco audacity.

We spoke to Mr Gross, an auto writer for more than 40 years and former director of the Petersen Automotive Museum in LA, about this priceless "kinetic art", how these beautiful cars came to be, and what they mean in contemporary culture. "The classic cars of the Art-Deco age remain today as among the most visually exciting, iconic and refined designs of the 20th century," he says.

There were 18 cars in Sensuous Steel – *which was your favourite?*
That's tough! The car that epitomises Art Deco is the 1937 Delahaye 135 MS Roadster by Figoni & Falaschi. I call it a "Paris gown on wheels". It's a feminine car, but underneath it has muscles. It's curvaceous, impractical, stunning from any angle. You *arrive* in that car.

What's the story behind it?
It was built as a one-off roadster for the 1937 Paris Auto Salon. It was stunning but also novel in terms of engineering – the

aerodynamics, special lightweight seats and the convertible top. It was purchased after the salon by the Ambassador of Brazil, but in 1939 a Frenchman bought it and stored it away on the Côte d'Azur until an Italian army officer took it. He fled the war and the original owner found it in Milan in 1947. He restored it at the Figoni workshop and the finishing trim touches were applied by Hermès. [US car connoisseur] Mr Miles Collier bought it in 2001 and restored it. The Collier Collection is one of the most important collections in the US – it houses everything from Porsches to Gary Cooper's Duesenberg.

What do you admire about Art-Deco design?
I love the simplicity of it. My friend Gary Vasilash [the editor of *Automotive Design & Production*] talks about the combination of fine lines and curves – which are both simple and complex. It's immediately recognisable. It's like the judge that was asked to define pornography. I can't define it, but I know it when I see it! These cars are kinetic art. Ralph Lauren's cars have been in the Louvre in Paris – people accept them as modern sculpture.

How do cars fit in among the general Art-Deco explosion during the 1920s and 1930s?
From 1930 to the outbreak of war in 1939, the Great Depression impacted. There were, however, people who could afford a special automobile. By 1937 and 1938, people felt the threat of war. It was a case of "let's enjoy this while we can". People would obtain a chassis from the factory and it was then taken to a coachbuilder; they looked at sketches and picked fabrics and leathers – the cars were bespoke.

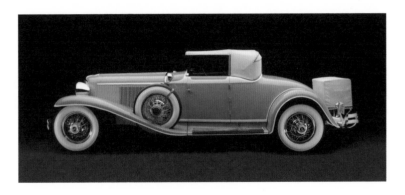

L-29 CORD CABRIOLET

Designed by Mr Alan Leamy, the L-29 Cord Cabriolet was the first US front-drive luxury car and represented a high watermark in Art-Deco influence. The marque's dramatically low silhouette appealed to its former owner, architect Mr Frank Lloyd Wright.

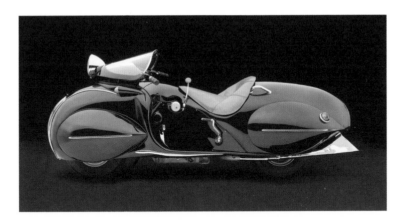

KJ HENDERSON WESTFALL

A rare example of 1930s motorcycle design, this aerodynamic two-wheeler was designed by Mr O Ray Courtney in 1936 as a "motorcycle of tomorrow". Running on an inline four cylinder, it was rebuilt by its current owner, Mr Frank Westfall.

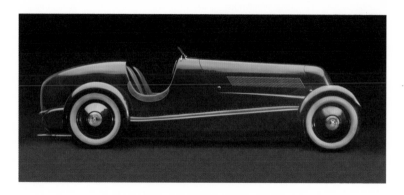

FORD MODEL 40 SPEEDSTER

Designed in 1932 by Ford's styling chief, Mr ET "Bob" Gregorie, the Speedster has a sleek two-seater aluminium body, with a streamlined chassis, curvaceous fenders, an alligator hood and a Ford flathead V8. It is the only one of its kind ever made.

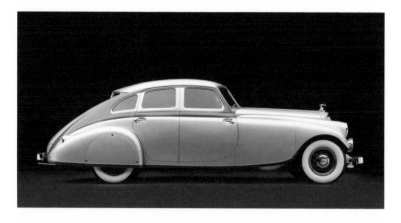

1934 PIERCE-ARROW SILVER ARROW SEDAN

The Arrow Sedan was originally built for the 1933 Chicago Century of Progress exposition. Designed by Mr Phillip Wright, this car epitomised luxury, with a price tag of $10,000 (roughly $170,000 today). Only three of the five of these made survive to this day.

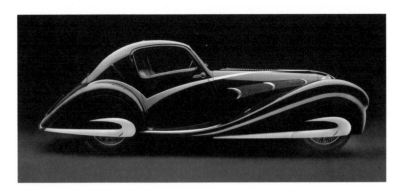

DELAHAYE 135 M

One of famed coachbuilder Mr Joseph Figoni's first aerodynamic coupé designs, the Delahaye 135 M was commissioned by French race car driver Mr Albert Perrot. It appeared at a *concours d'élegance* in Cannes in the 1930s, where it won the Grand Prix event.

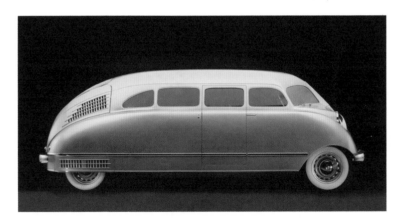

1935 STOUT SCARAB

With his extensive aeronautical background, Mr William "Bill" Bushnell Stout's Art-Deco-style 1935 Stout Scarab, which calls to mind the fuselage of a passenger plane, offered a roomy compartment – indeed, Mr Stout envisaged his design as an office on wheels.

Were these cars prime examples of their day?
Yes. They were expensive and exclusive, with technical innovations. The Pierce-Arrow Silver Arrow sedan won the 1933 Chicago Century of Progress exposition. The fenders are completely enveloped. Instead of the spares being out on the running board, they are hidden under the fenders. It amazed people. The Chrysler Airflow – that was almost too advanced. People didn't want their cars to look like a teardrop.

The 1934 Edsel Ford Model 40 Speedster is the only one of its kind. Who owns it and how much would it fetch?
When Mr Edsel Ford [the son of Mr Henry Ford] died in 1943 it was sold as part of his estate to owners in California. Edsel & Eleanor Ford House purchased the car for more than $1.3m in 2010 and spent a lot of money restoring it. It'd be north of $5m at auction.

Do you have any other interesting stories?
The Bugatti type 57C was a wedding gift from the government of France to the Prince of Persia – to keep that oil flowing! In 1930, people were interested in the Jordan Model Z Speedway Ace roadster, but the Depression had hit. I wrote an article in the 1970s saying that it had gone forever, but a man called Mr Jim Stecker who lived in Cleveland read that article, found the car and restored it. I've never been so glad to be wrong. The 1929 Cord L-29 Cabriolet was owned by architect Mr Frank Lloyd Wright. He thought the architecture of the Cord – a front-wheel drive with a low silhouette – complemented his buildings.

What attracts you to automobiles?
I bought my first issue of *Road & Track* when I was 12 years old. My neighbour had a sporty MG TC, which I loved – it wasn't a "turgid, jelly-bodied clunker" like writer Mr Ken Purdy's description of US cars. Recently, I drove a Cord 812 Convertible coupé from Virginia to Auburn, Indiana, where they were made.

It's wonderful to be in an old car. Your mind goes back in time – the smells, air changes and mechanicalness of the shifting gears.

What cars do you own?

I had two Ferraris and a Lamborghini, but now I have a garage filled with vintage Fords, including a 1939 convertible coupé and a 1940 coupé. I used to work on them when I was in high school. I have a 1932 Ford Roadster, which is quite a hot rod. I love the opportunity to drive old cars – it's like a pilot with his logbook. The leather, wood construction and ambience is totally different from a modern car. You have to get into a mind-set too – these cars won't stop in time!

How does the construction of cars then compare to now?

It's almost totally different. There were no safety regulations – nothing about emissions in the 1930s. A designer was free to do as he pleased. A lot of these cars are svelte; the tyres are thin. Modern cars have wider wheels to accommodate the likes of disc brakes.

Do you think we'll feel the same nostalgia about contemporary cars?

We'll never see cars like these again, but there are certain cars today that are exciting – Ferraris, Lamborghinis, Aston Martins. They really perform. You couldn't have imagined more than 500bhp back then. But the utilitarian cars, I don't think so. It won't be the same.

Do Art-Deco cars influence modern ones?

Designers today love to look to the past for styling cues – the roof lines, for example. The 1934 Type 46 Bugatti has a radical windshield and a perfect curve that runs over the top. You'll find that same line on some modern cars of the past 10 or 15 years. People love that purity of form.

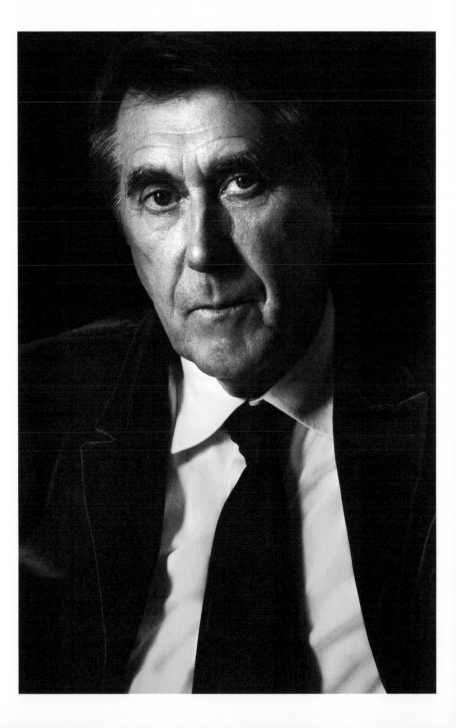

THE INTERVIEW

MR BRYAN FERRY

*The languorous legend talks jazz, the 1920s
and wearing hats in Paris*

Words by Mr Dan Cairns

EACH TIME I meet Mr Bryan Ferry, I itch to ask him a certain question. Not about his music – which he has been bewitching and beguiling us with for 40 years now, a milestone the singer celebrated with the release of *The Jazz Age*, an album of new versions of his songs, both Roxy Music and solo, retooled as lost classics from the Roaring Twenties. No, the question I always intend – and, hopelessly fail – to ask Mr Ferry is about a particular colour, and its key, but infinitesimally subtle, variations. For this is a man whose everyday wear will, more often than not, feature a navy suit, a matching tie, and a shirt of the palest blue. But not any old navy, or any old pale blue. That's the point. And I want that suit, that tie, and I want that shirt, too – and I want to ask Mr Ferry where I can find them. You see, his suits and ties are in a navy that is never merely dark blue yet isn't quite black, either. Similarly, his shirts are neither precisely white, nor verging on grey: they contain a passing hint of blue – barely there, but sartorially just so. The combination is, on Mr Ferry, always, always, a maddeningly immaculate one.

Predictably, when we meet again – amid the aptly restrained and nonchalant elegance of the Home House private members club in central London – I again fail to ask Mr Ferry about the colour blue. (I suspect I remain tongue-tied because I cannot bear the thought of him gazing down from those lazy eyelids, an expression of pity on his face, as if to say: "You mean you don't know?") I ask him, instead, about *The Jazz Age*, and the period in the 20th century after which the album is named.

A man whose attention to detail borders on the obsessive – "Oh, it does," Mr Ferry chuckles, "but it's an approved obsession, if you like" – was always going to pay attention to an album sleeve. The cover images and artwork for all of his releases seem to have gone through some sort of rigorous taste test before passing muster, and so it proves with *The Jazz Age*. Featuring a detail from *Le Tumulte Noir* series by the renowned French poster artist (and lover of singer, dancer and actress Ms Josephine Baker) Mr Paul Colin, it encases a sequence of songs that slip gracefully and evocatively into a big-band jazz setting: "Love is the Drug" becomes an even woozier and more louche affair than the original recording; "Do the Strand" a sort of narcotised Charleston; while dovetailing woodwind makes "Avalon" somehow even more forlorn than before. Crucially, if surprisingly, Mr Ferry has elected not to sing on the album, which is entirely instrumental. Was he never tempted to amble up to the vocal booth?

"Well, there was a bit of pressure to do so," he replies, with a wry laugh, "or insinuations, at least. You know, 'Couldn't you sing on, maybe, one of them?' But the whole point of the project was to see how well the songs could stand up without words, and to put the spotlight, as it were, on the part of me that is a songwriter, rather than the guy who stands on stage with a microphone." The decision to locate the new album in the 1920s was not one, Mr Ferry admits, that he could have imagined making before. "If you'd told me 20 years ago I'd be doing this, I'd have laughed. Although I was a big jazz fan as a young lad, once rock'n'roll came into my life and took it over, I pretty much stopped listening to it. I'd been seduced, carried off by wah-wah pedals and the sound of the electric guitar." He was drawn back to the 1920s, he says, because "it's such a fascinating period – the beginning of modernism. Eliot wrote *The Waste Land*, Scott Fitzgerald celebrated the period in *The Great Gatsby*. Reading that novel was my first introduction to that age, and he was the first writer I took to as a fan of literature. I mean, I'd been forced to read Milton and Shakespeare and everything else at school, but to read for pleasure was like, 'Whoa – this is the beginning of something.' I had this amazing sense of discovery." Does he ever feel as if he was born at the wrong time? "Well, Paris, Berlin, New York in the 1920s, there was so much going on. However, we don't live then, we live now. People say to me, 'Don't you wish you lived in the 1920s?', and I always go, 'No, not really.' I like the fact that I can get on a train to Paris, or fly to Berlin, and be there in two hours. It must have been fabulous to be around then, though. For a start, everyone wore hats. I don't tend to wear a hat in London, because I don't like being recognised, and people tend to [notice you] here if you wear one. I can get away with one in Paris, because it's more flamboyant there."

Mr Ferry was at the beginning of something himself, of course: it is impossible not to now view the period at the dawn of the 1970s – when acts such as Roxy Music and Mr David Bowie bade adieu to the previous decade and strode forth in a blaze of eyeliner, bombastic art-pop, outrageous but sharply design-savvy stage outfits and bold album imagery – as anything other than revolutionary (and, yes, liberatingly flamboyant). In Mr Ferry's case, however, there was always, alongside the restless trailblazing, a contrasting languor that was almost ennui, and a keening for more old-fashioned notions of elegance and sophistication: witness his tuxedo on the sleeve of his second solo album, 1974's *Another Time, Another Place*; his definitive and ineffably languid 1973 cover version of "These Foolish Things"; Mr Nicky Haslam's acute, long-ago remark that the singer would be more likely to redecorate a hotel room than wreck it; and Mr Ferry's film-star poise every time he looked at the camera, a cigarette curled between his fingers. The cigs may have gone now, but that look is still there. And, if the pace of change has slowed for Mr Ferry in the ensuing years, as it has for many of his contemporaries, he remains a man of boundless curiosity, still a "taste tarantula" (in the words of his old friend, the designer Mr Antony Price), still collecting, dissecting, sifting and, yes, redecorating – for what else is *The Jazz Age* but an exercise in immaculate rearrangement?

"When I'm writing a song," Mr Ferry says, as we conclude the interview, "I'm very much on my own. That first stage is a kind of lonely one, where you're wrestling with your demons, or however you care to phrase it, or looking for something new to say. Most of the time you're just thinking, 'Is this any good? Is this any different to what I've done before?'" Well, *The Jazz Age* is better than good, and it's certainly different.

Mr Ferry gets up to leave. Did I forget to mention what he's wearing? Oh, only a suit and tie of the most unimpeachable navy blue. And that pale, pale shirt. Damn the man.

ACKNOWLEDGEMENTS

Editor-in-Chief – Mr Jeremy Langmead
Creative Director – Mr Leon St-Amour
Editor – Ms Jodie Harrison
Production Director – Ms Xanthe Greenhill
Style Director – Mr Dan May
Designer – Mr Eric Åhnebrink
Chief Sub-Editor – Ms Siân Morgan
Deputy Sub-Editor – Mr James Coulson
Picture Editor – Ms Katie Morgan
Editorial Assistant – Ms Caroline Hogan

CONTRIBUTORS

Ms Marie Belmoh, Mr Rik Burgess, Mr Jacopo Maria Cinti,
Mr Tony Cook, Ms Iona Davies, Mr Chris Elvidge,
Mr Mansel Fletcher, Mr Tom M Ford, Mr Patrick Guilfoyle,
Ms Sophie Hardcastle, Mr Tom Harris, Mr Peter Henderson,
Mr Lewis Malpas, Mr David Pearson, Ms Rachael Smart,
Mr Scott Stephenson, Mr Ian Tansley, Mr Angelo Trofa

With thanks to
Ms Natalie Massenet

CREDITS

MR PORTER is the global online retail
destination for men's style,
offering more than 200 of the world's
leading menswear brands.

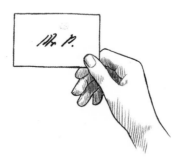